Dr Kate Gregorevic is a geriatrician and internal medicine physician. She works in both acute hospital medicine and community settings. She has also completed a PhD looking at the impact of positive psychosocial factors in the development of frailty in older adults. She has published multiple studies in this area.

Lifestyle medicine is a core feature of Kate's clinical practice, and nutrition, exercise and sleep are integral to developing plans to optimise her patients' health. Her approach goes beyond physical, by working with people to identify their own priorities and values, and always centring these in any management plans.

Kate feels that it is incredibly important to provide accurate lifestyle strategies for health to as many people as possible, so she has been published extensively, including *Sydney Morning Herald*, *The Age*, news.com.au, WHIMN and Mamamia. She has been heard on ABC breakfast radio and 3AW.

Kate is also the director of Project Three Six Twelve, an online wellbeing and exercise program giving women over 40 the tools they need to improve strength and vitality.

Kate lives in Melbourne with her husband and three children.

STAYING ALIVE

DR KATE GREGOREVIC

SPECIALIST AUSTRALIAN GERIATRICIAN AND
INTERNAL MEDICINE PHYSICIAN

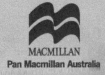

MACMILLAN
Pan Macmillan Australia

We advise that the information contained in this book does not negate personal responsibility on the part of the reader for their own health and safety. It is recommended that individually tailored advice is sought from your healthcare or medical professional. The publishers and their respective employees, agents and authors, are not liable for injuries or damage occasioned to any person as a result of reading or following the information contained in this book.

Some of the people in this book have had their names changed to protect their identities.

First published 2020 in Macmillan by Pan Macmillan Australia Pty Ltd
1 Market Street, Sydney, New South Wales, Australia, 2000

Cataloguing-in-Publication entry is available
from the National Library of Australia
http://catalogue.nla.gov.au

Typeset in 11/17 pt Sabon by Post Pre-press Group
Printed and bound in Australia by Ive Group

Any health or medical content contained in this book is not intended as health or medical advice. The publishers and their respective employees, agents and authors are not liable for injuries or damage occasioned to any person as a result of reading or following any health or medical content contained in this book.

The author and the publisher have made every effort to contact copyright holders for material used in this book. Any person or organisation that may have been overlooked should contact the publisher.

Aboriginal and Torres Strait Islander people should be aware that this book may contain images or names of people now deceased.

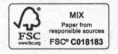

MIX
Paper from
responsible sources
FSC® C018183

The paper in this book is FSC certified.
FSC promotes environmentally responsible,
socially beneficial and economically viable
management of the world's forests.

To my husband and children,
my best reasons for staying alive

CONTENTS

INTRODUCTION

Living as long as possible shouldn't come at the expense of enjoying the present.

One of the greatest gifts of being a doctor for older adults is the constant reminder that life is fragile, finite and precious. This makes me want to protect my life and my health because I want to live as long and as well as possible, but it also reminds me to enjoy today, in case that is all there is.

The competing knowledge that our lifestyle choices can prolong life, but that death is also inevitable can present one of the most challenging conflicts of human existence. It manifests in the small, everyday decisions we make. Will I eat this piece of cake now: the delicious taste versus the longer-term risk of diabetes? Will I have another glass of wine: the light-headed buzz versus the increased risk of cancer? Will I go to bed or just stream another episode of a gripping TV show: the entertainment now or decreasing my risk of dementia with adequate sleep?

I regularly have the privilege of looking after people who have lived eight or nine decades. It is incredible to discover the wisdom and perspective that comes from living an incredibly long life.

For so many of my patients, there is also a recognition that time has become something concrete and measured; with most of their years behind them there is a deep insight of what truly matters in life.

Age is not a number

As a geriatrician, most of my patients have problems related to age. This does not mean they are all 'old'. There can be vast disparities in health between two people of the same age. My own grandmother has the kind of life that many of us aspire to enjoy in their nineties: she lives independently, tends her garden, walks her dog and is on the board of a charity. I see others who are living lives far more constrained by physical or cognitive impairments – some in their sixties and seventies needing carers on hand at all times.

While one of the best ways to reach very old age is to choose your parents wisely, for most of us, the number of healthy years lived will be influenced by our lifestyle choices. While people love to tell stories of people who lived to ninety while smoking a packet of cigarettes a day, these people are memorable in their rarity. Those who died young of smoking-related illness are no longer here to tell their story.

The traditional medical model of health is defined as the absence of disease by avoiding risk factors. It wasn't until I started my PhD research, exploring a framework of health outside this traditional model, that I truly understood that there is no conflict between the way we feel today and doing the best for our future. I discovered another framework for health, one that focuses on creating health by including positives, rather than avoiding negatives.

It was my PhD supervisor, Professor Ruth Hubbard, who first suggested looking at positive factors associated with recovery rather than negatives. These are called health assets, factors that are desirable in their own right that are also associated with the creation of wellbeing. This approach is based on an idea with the lovely name 'salutogenesis', a word coined by sociologist Aaron Antonovsky. Salutogenesis is a theory of health that posits that we and our communities have resources that we can use to optimise our wellbeing, and that these are desirable in their own right. Basically, including more things that improve life today is a strategy to increase longevity. This concept of health also goes beyond the idea that health is purely physical; it also incorporates social and mental health, as well as the concept of happiness.

Live for today, not just tomorrow

In my clinical work and through my research I have been able to explore some of the key factors that influence health and wellbeing in old age. Indeed, when I meet people and they find out what I do, I am often asked for advice on how to achieve longevity. This is perfectly understandable, especially when you consider that there are thousands of studies showing the benefits of lifestyle in achieving longevity, but we need to put this in context – despite numerous eminent researchers working to unlock the secrets of ageing, no one has ever made it stop; no one has ever solved the problem of death.

We rarely allow ourselves to think this overwhelming thought, but for every single one of us, life is fragile and uncertain. Even following all the right advice, we could develop an incurable disease tomorrow or even die suddenly today. This is why the question of how to live well today is so urgent: we need to start thinking about what makes life worthwhile in the present.

Most of us will have goals we are working towards – biggerpicture goals that are important for our sense of self and that create structure in our lives – but it is the day-to-day minutiae that makes a life. It is discovering a new and delicious food, going out for a walk and seeing the morning light reflecting on a building or running into an old, much-loved friend.

Living well means creating the right conditions to feel positive, energetic and engaged. And that does not mean always taking the easiest option – making the choice to feel better can be effortful, especially if it means a change in habits.

The secret to longevity

If you are looking for a simple, rigid solution to longevity, this is the wrong book. There is no one best life that will suit every person – only you can define this for yourself. Instead, I hope to empower you with the knowledge to create your own framework so you can live your own best life, starting today.

In the first part of the book, I will explain what happens as we age – not the external changes that we all see, but the changes that occur at the DNA and cellular level. These changes have their basis in the cellular processes that are inevitable for life. These changes don't occur at the same linear rate in everybody, and they are influenced by many factors in life.

Ageing is also associated with key changes in the way our immune systems work, called inflammaging. Put very simply, in people who are frail and older, the immune system is both more active and less efficient. These cellular and immune changes translate to changes in how our bodies work, and this can lead to frailty.

In part 2, I show you how the day-to-day lifestyle choices you make can not only improve your physical and mental health in the present but also affect cellular ageing and decrease the risk of chronic disease, frailty and dementia. This section looks at nutrition in healthy ageing, movement, and how sleeping well, being cognitively challenged, having plenty of social connections and feeling a sense of purpose all influence the rate of ageing.

Yet it is an inescapable truth that with age comes an increased risk of developing a chronic disease. Almost everyone I speak to who is aged over 50 has something like high blood pressure, or has had some sort of medical event, perhaps just the removal of a precancerous mole. Even if these health conditions don't kill us (and many won't), they can make life a lot less enjoyable. In part 3 I go into more detail about some of these conditions, including heart disease, stroke, dementia and frailty. Recognising the symptoms of these conditions is important, so you can get medical help. But I also want you to remember that almost all of these conditions share the same underlying causes. This is why prevention is such an excellent all-for-one deal!

This book isn't just about eating and exercise. Although they are important, health in humans goes beyond the physical. We have the most incredible capacity for thought, creativity and love, and these are all part of health. One thing I have learnt from my patients is that it is almost impossible to make positive changes for physical health without first feeling like your life matters. Creating purpose and having emotional connection with other people are integral components of health, and I see these as the foundations for making positive change.

My approach is not about denying enjoyment, it is about creating vitality so we can enrich our lives and live with meaning and engagement.

Our days are full of small decisions: What will I make for dinner? Will I walk or drive? Will I see if my friend is free for coffee? While they may seem minor, it's these decisions that accumulate over time to contribute to our future health. They also affect how well we feel today – our sleep, our mood, our energy levels. These decisions require us to prioritise our own health and wellbeing – which can be a challenge for many people

There are important factors in expected gender roles that also influence ageing. Women often take on more hours of caring than men, both for children and older relatives. Although caring for others can be enriching and rewarding, if it is constant and unrelenting it can have negative implications for health. Many women will spend decades creating favourite meals for loved ones, but would never take the time to make something special for themselves. Similarly, women are less likely than men to undertake regular exercise; many feel self-conscious and fear being judged, missing out on the immediate and long-term health benefits.

Men are more likely to engage in risky behaviours and to use higher levels of drugs and alcohol, perhaps as a response to rigid tropes of masculinity, where they are discouraged from expressing negative emotions.

I have written this book to show you that we all have the capacity to create health with our own strengths and resources. Making day-to-day decisions that optimise a feeling of wellness today ensures that our finite days are as satisfying as possible, with the excellent happenstance of longevity.

PART 1
UNDERSTANDING AGEING

WHAT IS A CELL?

Cells are the building blocks that make up all living things. All living organisms, other than single-cellular ones like bacteria, are made up of cells working together. Even within the human body, where all our cells have the same DNA, or coding instructions, they can look very different from each other and perform very different functions.

Each cell has its own semi-permeable membrane, which keeps the inside of the cell separate from its surrounding environment. Cells need to maintain the right mix of water and chemicals within them, but they also need to take in nutrients and oxygen and release any waste products or functional molecules they have produced. Their semi-permeable cell membrane makes this possible.

Our cells vary hugely in shape and internal function depending on their location and job. Muscle cells in our quadriceps are shaped like tubes, with proteins that can shorten and lengthen to allow the muscle to contract and relax. Our gut cells are covered in tiny finger-like projections, which increase their surface area and optimise absorption of gut nutrients. Skin cells are flat and layered on top of each other to form a protective barrier. White blood cells travel around the body in blood and change shape when they encounter a pathogen so they can ingest and kill it. These different shapes all result from expression of different genes, and they all have an essential role.

WHAT IS INSIDE A CELL?

Cells contain special structures called organelles. Different organelles perform specific functions, but work together in a synchronised way, like a production line in a factory.

The nucleus – this contains the cell's DNA, which is housed inside a special membrane that permits certain small molecules in and out. The DNA needs to be protected because it contains the instructions that make cells. DNA expression is tightly regulated to control which proteins are made.

The cytoskeleton – this is an internal framework that helps the cell maintain its shape and provides the mechanical support that cells need to perform their functions. In some cells these filaments can slide against each other, enabling the cells to move.

The mitochondria – these organelles use oxygen to make energy available for chemical reactions within cells. These organelles most likely originated over a billion years ago as bacteria that were engulfed by another cell. Instead of being digested, they continued living inside the cell and came to perform a critical function. Mitochondria also contain some of their own DNA, and are inherited exclusively from the mother via the ovum. They can also divide independently in response to the cell's energy demands.

The endomembrane system – this system facilitates the production and transfer of cell membranes and is made up of multiple components: the **endoplasmic reticulum (ER)**, **Golgi apparatus** and **lysosomes**. The endoplasmic reticulum is a system of membranes involved in protein synthesis. The Golgi apparatus is part of the production line for proteins, where the sequence of amino acids undergoes folding and packaging for delivery to its target destination. Lysosomes break down molecules so their parts can be recycled. These membranes are contiguous with each other, and substances move between them in **vesicles**, which are small bubbles surrounded by membranes within the cell.

1

LIFE EXPECTANCY

That most babies born today will live for nine decades is
truly one of humanity's greatest successes.

It is only relatively recently that enough people have actually reached old age to enable us to study why and how some people stay healthy while others die young. In 1900, the worldwide average life expectancy was 31 years; now it is 71 years, and in developed countries like Japan, the UK and Australia it is over 80.

This change is largely the result of improvements in public health, such as clean water and better nutrition, which has a huge impact, particularly at the start of life. In the UK in 1850, 15 per cent of babies died in their first year, largely due to poor sanitation and preventable disease. These staggeringly high infant and child mortality rates substantially decreased the average life expectancy figure. Fast-forward 160 years and infant mortality is now 0.38 per cent in the UK and 0.31 per cent in Australia.

For women, this improvement in life expectancy is in no small part due to better obstetric care and greater control over their own fertility. My own grandmother had a placenta that was lying over her cervix, meaning it was impossible for her baby to be born vaginally, which was undetectable in the days before ultrasound. When she began haemorrhaging in early labour, an emergency caesarean stopped her from bleeding to death and she and my aunt were saved. Today, this problem would have been identified on ultrasound and the operation safely planned, further reducing the risk to mother and baby.

The gains in life expectancy have also derived from better management of medical conditions that were previously immediately fatal. Heart failure, diabetes and kidney disease are among the many chronic diseases that people can now live with for many years. My great, great grandfather died in 1908, aged 40, from type 1 diabetes, where the immune system attacks the pancreas and stops insulin production. Despite being described in his obituary as the physical embodiment of robust health, he became unwell on a Wednesday and died that Saturday from a diabetic coma. If this happened to a 40-year-old now, they would simply start injecting insulin. Instead of a death sentence, diabetes is now a chronic disease, managed with medication and diet. Living with type 1 diabetes requires vigilance – too little insulin can lead to long-term organ damage, too much can cause hypoglycaemia – but I have met people in their eighties who have worked with their doctor to successfully negotiate this disease for decades, maintaining excellent health.

Yet one of the most seismic contributions to our increased life expectancy is something so routine that we don't even consider it a major scientific advance. Every year we are encouraged to visit our family doctor to have our blood pressure, cholesterol, diet and blood sugar checked. And the reason we do this can be traced back to the Framingham Heart Study. In 1948, researchers recruited 5209 people from the town of Framingham in the USA to examine mortality and heart disease. Every two years, the dedicated study participants provided dietary information, smoking status and medical records and undertook blood tests as well as having their weight, height and blood pressure measured. They even participated in cognitive assessments and provided personal information about things like employment and education. Researchers soon had evidence that smoking, obesity, elevated cholesterol and blood pressure increased the risk of heart disease, and that exercise decreased it.

Similar longitudinal population studies, such as the Nurses' Health Study (begun in the 1970s) and the Physicians' Health Study (begun in the 1980s) have also been invaluable in identifying the risk factors for heart disease, stroke and cancer. These studies are ongoing; the Framingham researchers have even recruited the children and some grandchildren of the original cohort.

That most babies born today will live for around nine decades is the culmination of thousands of small and large scientific discoveries and is truly one of humanity's greatest successes.

The 'ageing population' is so often framed as a negative, but the reality is that *we* are the ageing population – every single one of us is getting older. Indeed, over the next 50 years the proportion of adults aged 65 and older is predicted to almost double, from 14 per cent to around 25 per cent of the population. As more people achieve a long life, the stereotype of people of 'advanced age' being fixed, staid and unchanging is being smashed. Inspirational people like actors Dame Judi Dench and Jane Fonda, writer Margaret Atwood, scientist Elizabeth Blackburn and TV-presenter-turned-activist Sir David Attenborough are living proof that we do not lose our intellectual drive or creativity as we enter old age. When most of us turn 60, we will have one-third of our lives left to live. That's three decades of opportunity to seek new experiences, forge new connections and enjoy every moment.

2

CELLULAR AGEING

Ageing, put simply, is the cumulative effect of changes in our cellular machinery that occur over time.

When we think of ageing, we often think of changes we can see, such as white hair, wrinkled skin or having to walk with a cane, but ageing is actually something that is happening at a microscopic level, related to cellular processes that start at conception. Every second, the trillions of cells that make up our bodies are undertaking the biochemical reactions that keep us alive: red blood cells are delivering oxygen; heart cells are contracting; pancreatic cells are secreting hormones to balance blood sugar; kidney cells are balancing the salts and acid in our blood; brain cells (neurons) are firing impulses that enable us to read and understand these words. All of these processes require energy, but this energy production damages our cells. Ageing, put simply, is the cumulative effect of changes in our cellular machinery that occur over time. Understanding these changes is the first step to ensuring that our lifestyle will enable us to enjoy good health for as long as possible.

DEOXYRIBONUCLEIC ACID (DNA)

'What did Watson and Crick discover?'

'Rosalind Franklin's notes.'

Although James Watson, Francis Crick and Maurice Wilkins won the Nobel prize for discovering the structure of DNA, they only did so after looking at Rosalind Franklin's notes, allegedly without her permission. When Watson and Crick wrote their paper, they even neglected to include her as an author. Rosalind Franklin died, aged 38, before the Nobel prize was awarded, but she should be remembered as one of the discoverers of the structure of DNA.

DNA, or deoxyribonucleic acid, is the incredible molecule that contains the instructions for all our cells. The sequence of chemical building blocks that codes for one set of instructions is called a gene. The information in DNA is translated into a sequence of amino acids, which can be translated into a protein. These proteins can be structural, chemical messengers, hormones or enzymes.

Since each one of our cells originated from that first fertilised ovum, they all contain exactly the same DNA. DNA enables life by being both a template for its own replication and providing the instructions to build lifeforms. If our body is hardware, the DNA is the software that tells it how to run. Our DNA is in the nucleus of the cell and forms chromosomes, or strands of DNA. The DNA has a backbone and each step is made of two paired nucleotides, which are sometimes called bases. There are four types of nucleotides: cytosine, thymine, adenine and guanine. Due to their chemical structure, cytosine pairs with guanine and adenine pairs with thymine, like puzzle pieces. This structure enables DNA to reproduce itself exactly because in reproduction, when the steps come apart, each backbone provides the template for a new strand.

Since each cell contains 2 metres of DNA, when our cells are not dividing, DNA is tightly wound into chromosomes. When a cell divides, the double helix unravels. Enzymes (helper proteins) in the cell then allow new nucleotides to join to their complementary base pairs, while another enzyme joins the backbone together, creating a strand of DNA identical to the original.

Our DNA is not just one long string. Each cell actually contains 46 chromosomes, or pieces of DNA. These comprise 23 pairs, with one chromosome from each parent. On each chromosome there are particular sequences of bases, called genes. Around 99.9 per cent of each person's DNA is the same.

Our cells change with age

The cells that make up our bodies are like a strong community – different cells have different roles, but they all depend on one another to thrive. For example, our skin cells form a barrier to the outside world, but they are dependent on gut cells digesting food for energy, heart cells for pumping blood and lung cells for exchanging oxygen and carbon dioxide. Each cell needs to stay in its own place and to be willing to die for the survival of the organism when its time comes. If one cell type starts growing without any restriction and grows in other places in the body, this can result in cancer. I talk more about cancer in chapter 20.

Errors in cell replication

Our bodies need constant repair and rejuvenation. This involves making new cells by cell division, which is the process of a cell replicating itself. One of the critical functions of replication is to make an exact copy of the DNA. The base pairs need to line up exactly to create new chromosomes that are identical to the original cell. The new copy of DNA should be identical to the mother cell, but there can be errors in the order of nucleotides. Sometimes the replication process will 'skip' a nucleotide, so every one afterwards will be out of order or, in extreme cases, the DNA strand can break completely.

Sometimes these mistakes have no consequences at all: even with the change, the protein that comes from that gene will still work perfectly well. But sometimes, that one small substitution can mean that the daughter cell has a gene that no longer functions, or that takes on a new and harmful function. Depending on the role of this gene, this can have significant consequences, including further DNA damage.

Many things can increase the rate of DNA damage, such as smoking, certain chemicals, sunlight and certain compounds in foods we eat. Of course, it isn't possible to avoid all sources of damage – we can't stay out of the sun forever, and it wouldn't be good for us anyway!

Although our cells have mechanisms for repair, these are not perfect. Over time we can accumulate populations of cells with errors, particularly where there is high cell turnover, such as in the oesophagus and among white blood cells. One study published in the *New England Journal of Medicine* looked at people with identifiable populations of abnormal white blood cells, called clonal haematopoiesis of indeterminate potential, or CHIP. The incidence of CHIP increases with age, and it also increases the risk of heart disease. This may partly explain why even without traditional risk factors, we still become more likely to get heart disease as we age.

Mitochondrial damage

Mitochondria are the powerhouses of the cell. This is where glucose and oxygen react to make Adenosine triphosphate (ATP), which is the form of energy that all of our cells can use. Although this process is highly controlled, it is not perfect. A by-product is reactive oxygen species (ROS) which can damage the DNA and the mitochondria themselves. If the mitochondria are damaged, they become less efficient at producing energy.

REACTIVE OXYGEN SPECIES

Our cells primarily release the energy they get from carbohydrates, fats and proteins through a process called aerobic respiration. This is a series of chemical reactions that takes place in the mitochondria.

One of the by-products of this process is reactive oxygen species, or free radicals. These are molecules that are chemically unstable and ready to react with anything nearby. This reaction can change the molecular structure of other chemicals in the cell, damaging them, which can affect DNA, the cell membrane or even the mitochondria themselves. These reactive oxygen species aren't all bad, they also have important roles in the cells and are actually used as part of our defences against infections. Our bodies have our own defences against reactive oxygen species, but if these get overwhelmed, this is called oxidative stress, and may be a key cause of DNA damage. A few years ago, consuming antioxidants was all the rage as an anti-ageing strategy. The idea was that these would mop up the ROS and decrease rates of cell damage, but in clinical trials they don't work.

Telomere shortening

Telomeres are specialised caps of DNA at the end of our chromosomes that keep them intact. They are important because the way our DNA replicates means it is not able to go to the very end of a chromosome, so a few base pairs are lost with each replication. The telomeres are repeats of DNA that are not essential for coding, so they can be sacrificed. Over the course of many replications, telomeres get shorter and shorter, until they reach a critical length and the cell stops replicating. In test tubes, scientists have been able to make these cells continue to replicate, and the result is that the DNA of daughter cells is full of errors.

We all have an enzyme called telomerase that can repair the end of telomeres. This is active in dividing cells, and is usually absent in other cell types. In studies of centenarians, greater telomere length is associated with increased years of healthy life. People who have been born with DNA errors that prevent effective telomere repair show increased rates of ageing.

Epigenetic ageing

Although the genes we inherit are a limiting factor in our health and longevity, our everyday actions can impact how those genes are expressed. Epigenetics is the study of how gene expression is altered by environmental factors such as nutrition, exercise, whether we drink or smoke etc. The environment we create for ourselves can also influence our metabolic pathways and affect the rate of cellular ageing.

A muscle cell looks and functions very differently to an immune cell, or a nerve cell or a skin cell. Each cell contains the same genes, but not all of these genes are switched on in each cell. Epigenetics refers to the expression of genes. This is influenced by many environmental factors, and can even be inherited to a degree. As an example, a baby born to a malnourished mother may have more 'thrifty' genes switched on. This is controlled by a process called methylation, where the genes get stuck down, so they can't be expressed. The pattern of DNA methylation changes with age, and using complex mathematical modelling, this has been utilised to develop a measure of biological age called Horvath's clock. This has been associated with some age-related conditions, but more research needs to be done before this can be used in clinical practice.

Protein degradation

Proteins are the products of genes. The sequence of DNA codes for a specific sequence of amino acids, which then fold in on each other to make a specific shape with a specific function. Proteins have a spectacular number of different roles in our body. Some examples are actin and myosin, which let our muscles contract, enzymes, which speed up chemical reactions, and many more.

Proteins are strings of specific amino acids, which fold into a three dimensional shape that is essential for their function, the way only a specific key can fit in a lock. The shape of the protein is determined by the chemical attraction between the amino acids, but these bonds are relatively weak, and can be affected by environmental factors like heat. An example is cooking an egg and seeing the protein-rich fluid around the yolk turn white.

The folding of proteins into their specific shape is guided by chaperone proteins. These also help maintain proteostasis, which means proteins maintaining their shape.

This proteostasis network is regulated by genetic, epigenetic and environmental factors and shares many of the same controls as ageing and development. It also requires energy to be produced by mitochondria, which, as we saw earlier, can also become damaged with age or cellular stress. Sometimes proteins can become damaged and misfolded, by heat, chemicals or ROS. Some of the misfolded proteins can be removed, but others can also aggregate and form clumps. Misfolded proteins, particularly if they clump together, have been linked to some of the most well-known age-related diseases, including Alzheimer's disease and Parkinson's disease. Like many of the other biological processes involved in ageing, the protein repair system can also be influenced by nutrition and other factors that promote oxidative stress.

Stem cell depletion

Most mature cells in our body have become so specialised to their particular job that they have lost the ability to divide, which is why the role of stem cells is so important. When a cell has matured into its specific role in the body, this usually means it loses its ability to divide. Most of these cells can't live forever, and can be damaged or wear out. Stem cells are special cells that can keep dividing to make more cells or, with the right cellular signals, become any kind of specialised cell.

Different tissue types have their own stem cells, constantly replacing cells that have passed their useful lifespan. The constant wear and tear they endure from travelling around the body means red blood cells are one cell type that needs to be constantly replaced.

Red blood cells (RBCs) have the job of carrying oxygen from the lungs to the tissues, then carrying carbon dioxide back to the lungs to be exhaled. Their journey from the lungs starts in the largest blood vessel in the body, the aorta, which then branches into smaller and smaller vessels (veins), until finally the RBCs squeeze along tiny vessels called capillaries one at a time, so they can supply every single cell in our bodies.

In order to carry as much oxygen and carbon dioxide as

possible, mature RBCs don't have a nucleus, which means they don't have the DNA required for replication. The damage RBCs suffer as they are shunted around and squeezed through capillaries means that, after about 120 days, they are broken down in the spleen and their components, such as iron, are recycled. As a result, there is a constant need for new RBCs, and this is met by stem cells. The stem cells for blood are in the bone marrow, which by adulthood is predominantly found in the pelvis and vertebrae (in childhood the bone marrow is more widespread and is also in the limbs). These stem cells are also used to create white blood cells (which help fight infection) and platelets (which help blood to clot).

While stem cells persist through life, with age their numbers reduce. This can occur because the stem cells have divided too many times and have short telomeres, or because they have accumulated DNA damage. Our bodies have good reason to stop these cells dividing; if these damaged cells keep dividing, they can cause cancer.

THE LINKS BETWEEN CANCER AND AGEING

Although it might seem counterintuitive, many of the same processes that lead to cancer also lead to ageing. In both cancer and ageing, there is genetic instability. It may be that some of the cellular features of ageing are a direct way to deal with damaged cells to prevent them developing into a cancer that threatens the survival of the organism.

Although physicians have known about cancer for millennia (the Egyptians described it in 1600 BCE and the Greek physician Hippocrates is credited with naming it in around 300 BCE), it is only very recently that we have been able to actually understand the DNA and cellular changes that lead to cancer. This was largely made possible thanks to an unwitting donation by a woman named Henrietta Lacks.

Henrietta Lacks was born in 1920 in Virginia, USA. Her family were poor and she started tobacco farming at an early age. Henrietta gave birth to her first child, fathered by her cousin, aged fourteen. Following the birth of another child, she and her cousin married and moved to Maryland. Four months after the birth of her fifth child, she was diagnosed with cervical cancer at Johns Hopkins, the only hospital that treated black people in Baltimore. Henrietta died less than one year after her cancer diagnosis.

Unbeknownst to Henrietta and her family, samples of her tumour were living on in the laboratory. Without obtaining consent, cells were taken from the tumour and cultured by oncologist George Otto Gey; this cell line was called HeLa. HeLa was the first cell line that survived in the laboratory for more than a few days, and has been used in countless experiments, continuing to this day. In an attempt to account for the ethical transgressions of times past, Henrietta's family now have input into use of the genetic sequence.

How our bodies deal with damaged cells

Since cellular ageing is unavoidable, our bodies need ways of dealing with damaged cells. If the cells are damaged enough, they will undergo apoptosis, a programmed cell death. Other cells will enter senescence, where they can no longer replicate but are still able to perform other critical functions.

Apoptosis

Apoptosis refers to a controlled, programmed cell death. Cells can also die by necrosis, which can occur when the cell becomes damaged, such as in the case of a burn, or as a result of lack of blood supply or a virus. In necrosis, the cell ruptures, spewing its contents out into its surrounds, which causes inflammation. In apoptosis, the cell breaks down in a controlled way, into small packages so it can be collected by the body's garbage collection. Apoptosis is a very important process, and one that is crucial in order for our bodies to function properly. It can occur in response to DNA damage or a cell being infected with a virus, and it is even part of embryonic development.

Senescence

Senescence comes from the same Latin root as the word senile. This makes senescent cells sound old and decrepit, but what it actually means is that the cell stops dividing permanently and takes on other functions. Senescent cells perform an important role in tissues by releasing locally active messengers that suppress tumours and encourage tissue repair.

Once a damaged cell has been created, whether by DNA damage, physical trauma, heat or cold, this can trigger the cell to become senescent. Senescent cells affect the immune system by releasing chemical messengers that influence the function of cells around them in a variety of ways. They can also cause other cells around them to become senescent, increasing the number of non-functioning cells in an organ.

Senescent cells accumulate as we age, so although they help prevent cancer, they can also be key drivers of age-related change. In fact, studies in genetically engineered mice have shown that giving drugs that clear senescent cells can increase healthy life span, and this is effective even in older mice. While there have been some similar studies on human tissues, we're a long way off having a tablet we can take. Intriguingly, a study in *Diabetes* in 2016 shows that exercise might help to reduce senescent cells. Now that's something we don't have to wait for.

WHY CAN'T WE JUST TAKE HUMAN GROWTH HORMONE?

Human growth hormone is produced by the pituitary gland and promotes the growth and strength of bone and muscle. Its levels are highest at puberty, then they gradually decrease as we age, becoming almost unmeasurable after age 60, which is called the somatopause. This reduction in growth hormone seems to play a critical role in the loss of muscle mass and increase in body fat that occurs with ageing.

In the 1990s, there was interest in the possibility of using human growth hormone to 'treat' ageing, but researchers soon found that this actually increased the risk of diabetes and other diseases. While some people continue to source human growth hormone, often over the internet, to increase lean muscle mass, the health risks are not worth the aesthetic benefits.

The effects of using growth hormone come, in part, from stimulating the liver to release IGF-1 (insulin-like growth factor 1), which can also independently stimulate muscle growth. Somewhat counterintuitively, it seems that *lower* levels of IGF-1 or cell receptors that are less sensitive to IGF-1 in adult life are associated with increased lifespan. Mice that have been bred to have a decreased sensitivity to

IGF-1 are resistant to diabetes and cancer, although much smaller than mice without this genetic alteration.

While it is not ethical to try to alter these genes in humans, there are some people living with a naturally occurring form of resistance to growth hormone. Some studies of centenarians have found that they are more likely to have gene variants that reduce IGF-1 signalling. There is also a genetic disorder called Laron syndrome, where people are born with two missing copies of a gene for the receptor for growth hormone, meaning that they are resistant to its effects. Of the 300 people in the world who have this disorder, one third live in Ecuador. They have an average height of 120 centimetres and are almost completely resistant to cancer, however they do not have an increased life expectancy.

We are not beholden to our genes

In terms of human history, it is only an incredibly recent phenomenon that most of us can now expect to reach very old age. This increase in life expectancy isn't genetic, it's due to scientific advances. These cellular processes that constitute ageing don't happen at the same rate in everyone, and are heavily influenced by our lifestyle.

One of the most striking things I've learnt about ageing is that we still have so much to learn about how and why it happens. This is an incredibly exciting area, and although there is unlikely to be a quick fix, the key lifestyle strategies relating to nutrition, exercise and cognitive and emotional health all have a real biological impact. In the coming chapters I will highlight what we already know works, along with new areas of research that may lead to key strategies in the future.

ANIMAL MODELS AND AGEING

Have you ever read a headline about an amazing new ageing treatment that could double life expectancy, only to find out it's referring to a worm? Given that humans live for up to 120 years and rats for only three (and some nematode worms only last around two weeks), it is much easier to study cellular ageing in animals, or even yeast, than in humans.

It is fascinating how much commonality there is in metabolic pathways from simple, unicellular organisms right up to humans. This is particularly true for pathways related to food scarcity and controlling rates of cell growth, cell repair and cell replication. This makes sense; DNA repair is something all organisms need to deal with, and all organisms are at risk of dying if their food runs out.

However, we need to extrapolate these studies with caution for a very important reason: we still don't really know what determines the lifespan of a particular species. We don't know why rats live for two to three years while similarly sized squirrels live for 25 years.

This extends to drugs that may have an anti-ageing effect in animals, which include metformin (a drug used for diabetes) and rapamycin (an immunomodulating drug used in organ transplants). Although these are exciting developments, there are countless therapies that have worked in animals but not humans. As a clinician, my first duty is to do no harm, so without trial data in humans, including safety, I will not be prescribing these for my patients.

3

AGEING AND THE
IMMUNE SYSTEM

Inflammation isn't just associated with disease, but with ageing itself – so much so that we call it 'inflammaging'.

Put in the simplest terms, our immune system identifies things that shouldn't be in our bodies and removes them. This includes everything from parasites to fungi, bacteria and viruses. The immune system is particularly concentrated at the sites where pathogens, or disease-causing organisms, are more likely to enter our bodies, such as the skin, airways and gut. The immune system also plays a critical role in identifying and repairing damaged tissue and looking for cancer cells. As we age, our immune system becomes less able to control infections.

A SURPRISINGLY COMMON DIAGNOSIS

One diagnosis I make a few times a year in my older patients is genital herpes, which is usually caused by a close viral relative of the cold sore virus. Often the patient has had

---

an ulcer or rash for a while, and no one has thought to do a viral swab because we tend to associate sexually transmitted infections with young people. Notwithstanding that age is not a barrier to sexual relationships, for most people, the virus has been with them for decades, lying dormant in nerve cells. Often when people first acquire the virus, they don't get any symptoms; it is only when they are older, and their immune system is less robust, that they might experience their first clinical symptoms.

How the immune system works

The immune system consists of physical barriers, proteins, chemicals, specialised cells and organs that function in two major branches: innate and adaptive.

The innate immune system

Can you think back to a time when you had some sort of infection on your skin? The skin would have been red, warm and painful. Most of these changes are driven by the innate immune system, our first line of response.

The innate immune system has three layers: physical barriers such as skin and mucous; secretions such as saliva and gastric acid; and many specific cells and proteins. As we will discuss in the next chapter, gut bacteria help to keep our intestinal wall healthy, which is important – 70 per cent of our immune system is in our gut. Our gut wall has many lymph nodes and a ready supply of white blood cells. This makes sense when you consider that pathogens like salmonella and cholera enter our system in the food we eat.

There are many different cell types involved in the innate immune system. Macrophages are large white blood cells that destroy bacteria by engulfing it. Neutrophils release substances that act as a net to catch bacteria; while mast cells release potent inflammatory substances into the tissues, which increase blood flow and make the blood vessels leaky, so immune cells and fluid can get out. When you have a red, itchy mosquito bite, that's your mast cells at work.

The innate immune system works by pattern recognition. Many of the cells of the innate immune system are the frontline patrollers, out looking for trouble. These cells, called macrophages and dendritic cells, are a type of white blood cell that look a little like blobs with tentacles. They have receptors on their cell membranes called toll-like receptors (TLRs). These are activated by molecules that are commonly present on foreign microbes, like bacteria and fungi. When TLRs detect a threat, they communicate using cytokines, which are chemical messengers that have local and systemic effects. One of the local responses is to increase blood flow to an infected area to assist in healing. The cytokines can also cause systemic effects of fever and fatigue, leaving us feeling like we need a nap.

Some cytokines increase the immune response, while others help it to switch off once the threat has passed. This is incredibly important; an overactive immune response can be fatal, such as anaphylactic shock.

The immune system also plays a critical role in wound healing and can be activated by tissue damage, which is the body's way of preparing for a potential infection if there is a breach in the skin. The innate immune system can even be triggered by our own infected or abnormal cells if they don't display certain identifying traits on their surface. Natural killer (NK) cells are like overzealous police who shoot anyone who fails to produce identification.

Since pathogenic bacteria can produce copies of themselves within 20–30 minutes, this rapid response is critical to surviving an infection. The innate immune system is powerful and fast acting, but responds to patterns rather than specific organisms.

Fortunately, we also have a second, more sophisticated line of defence: the adaptive immune system.

The adaptive immune system

While the innate immune system mounts an instantaneous response to a threat, the adaptive immune system takes days to weeks, but results in a targeted response and sustained protection by making a 'memory' of the pathogen that can last a lifetime.

Dendritic cells are the key to communication between the innate and adaptive immune systems. These are found anywhere where the body is exposed to the external environment, like the skin or gut. When dendritic cells encounter a pathogen, they engulf it, then head back to headquarters: the lymph nodes. Lymph nodes are collections of immune tissue that are found in many places in the body (if you have ever had a sore throat and felt swollen tender lumps under your neck, these are lymph nodes). Once the dendritic cells get to the lymph nodes, they show the foreign invader to the B and T lymphocytes that live there, which then stimulate the production of antibodies. The lymphocytes secrete these antibodies into the blood and the extra-cellular fluid that bathes our cells, where they can latch on to the invaders and neutralise them, ready for them to be mopped up by macrophages.

These antibodies can also be secreted onto epithelial surfaces, like the airways in the lung or the gut, and into body fluids, notably breastmilk, which is why breastfeeding can help protect babies from infection. Once the threat is over, a few of these immune cells remember the invader, ready to attack at a moment's notice if it shows up again. This is why we can develop immunity to a previous infection, and why a vaccination can provide lifelong protection from a particular disease.

WHY DOESN'T THE IMMUNE SYSTEM JUST STAY 'ON'?

Since the dawn of life, fighting off invasion from microbes has been a constant threat. It is only incredibly recently in human history that infection has stopped being a major cause of death, particularly for babies and children. Without an immune system, human life simply isn't possible. So why doesn't it just stay 'on' all the time? Not only does mounting an immune response use significant energy and resources, an overactive immune system is also associated with tissue damage, which is why there are immune cells and cytokines whose job it is to help turn it down. When the checks and balances go wrong, people can develop an autoimmune disease. Sometimes this can mean that the body makes antibodies against our own tissues and destroy them and can occasionally be fatal.

Inflammation, chronic disease and ageing

When you have the flu, the virus is actually infecting the airways. Yet we experience muscle aches, fever, tiredness and lethargy. This is because of systemic inflammation. When the innate immune cells detect a dangerous invader, they release cytokines to activate the whole body's defences. A fever is a good example of this. The cytokines produced by the local immune cells travel through the blood to the hypothalamus in the brain and cause an increase in the set point for body temperature, which is why we shiver and feel cold when we have a fever. This actually helps to fight infection, because it makes bacterial growth less efficient. Cytokines also lead to illness behaviour, like wanting to crawl under a blanket and go to sleep.

Since any microbial threat can be deadly, cytokines activate components of the immune system and defences throughout the whole body, which is called systemic inflammation. Although this can be a marker of infection, it is also a response to many other things, such as certain cancers or environmental factors.

C-reactive protein (CRP), which is made in the liver in response to immune activation, is a marker of systemic inflammation that can be measured in the blood. Research has linked higher levels of systemic inflammation to atherosclerosis, a chronic, low-grade inflammation of the arterial wall. In atherosclerosis, there is a gradual accumulation of 'lipoproteins', fatty molecules, in the arterial wall. This activates macrophages, and the subsequent inflammation calls other types of inflammatory cells to the area. Muscle cells in the walls of the artery also take up the lipoproteins and can convert to macrophage-like cells.

A key part of inflammation is that it 'turns off', but in established atherosclerosis, there is an imbalance between the off signals and on signals, so the inflammatory process remains active and actually results in tissue damage. Over time, some of the macrophages become overwhelmed and die, forming a necrotic centre of the atherosclerotic plaque. This makes the plaque unstable and prone to rupture, which sets off a clotting cascade that can completely block the artery, which is what happens in a heart attack. The build-up of atherosclerosis takes decades, and the earliest changes can be seen in adolescence. Eating a diet high in omega-3 can help to decrease this process.

Inflammation isn't just associated with disease, but with ageing itself – so much so that we call it 'inflammaging'. Many older adults will have measurably higher levels of immune activity even though they do not have an infection. One theory is that the accumulation of damaged cells could be driving increased inflammation. As we saw in the previous chapter, senescent cells release a variety of pro-inflammatory signals, partly to suppress cancer. Damaged mitochondria are also powerful drivers of the innate immune system. Chronic infection, such as HIV, is also associated with earlier age-related changes.

One of the most difficult things to work out is whether inflammation represents the chicken or the egg. Some would argue that higher levels of inflammation directly damage tissue and drive the ageing process, while others argue that inflammation is simply a marker of age-related degeneration. Like many things in biology, this is complex and difficult to unpack. I suspect it is likely to be both, but we will have to wait and see what future research shows.

OBESITY AND METAFLAMMATION

In evolutionary history, there have been far stronger selective pressures to cope with food scarcity and starvation than the surfeit of kilojoules in wealthy, developed countries. While overeating, rather than starving, presents no immediate threat to health, our bodies have simply not evolved to live in an environment where it is a constant effort not to overeat.

One of the biggest health changes over recent decades has been the increasing number of people who are over-weight or obese. Obesity is defined as having a body mass index (BMI) of over 30, and has been linked with many illnesses, including diabetes, dementia, heart disease and lung disease. (BMI is calculated by dividing your weight in kilograms by your height in metres squared.) People who are obese are also at increased risk of frailty.

However, where fat is stored is also important. We know that fat carried around the abdomen is most highly associated with the development of disease. Abdominal fat has a greater number of senescent cells, which release proinflammatory cytokines. This may be because the high demand for fat storage leads to cell damage. In one animal experiment, mice were fed the 'mouse equivalent' of a human diet of highly processed foods and developed both obesity and higher levels of senescent cells. (Interestingly, exercise could reverse both these changes.) Of course, these are difficult experiments to conduct in humans, as it would be quite unethical to feed a human enough to deliberately induce obesity, and we still don't have reliable ways to measure cellular senescence in living people.

Metaflammation is the intersection between metabolism, or using energy, and inflammation. There are many ways that our immune system can be 'switched on'. Even eating can increase immune activation (this doesn't mean you should stop eating!). This makes good evolutionary sense, since it is possible to ingest harmful pathogens with a meal.

It seems likely that abdominal fat tissue drives inflammation by causing hormonal and cytokine changes. Similar to atherosclerosis, the uptake of fatty acids by macrophages turns them on to a pro-inflammatory state. Along with the adipose tissue itself, other factors trigger immune overactivation, such as food types, particularly ultra-processed foods, and inactivity. Like many things in human biology, it probably works both ways.

Slowing inflammaging

The regulation of the immune system is extremely complex and is influenced by multiple pathways in other bodily systems, including the digestive, circulatory and nervous systems. The same cytokines can stimulate (up-regulate) or suppress (down-regulate) the immune system depending on what is going on with the rest of the body. A good example is sauna use. In Finland, where most houses have a sauna, increased sauna use has been linked with protection against Alzheimer's disease and cardiovascular disease. When people heat up, they release a pro-inflammatory cytokine called IL-6. If this is released in the context of infection, it is pro-inflammatory. In the context of sauna, or exercise, however, it encourages the immune system to quickly turn off again. Almost all lifestyle interventions that influence the rate of cellular ageing will influence immune activity, and this is one of the most powerful pathways to improving wellbeing and longevity that we have.

BRUSH YOUR TEETH TO LIVE LONGER

We all know we are supposed to brush our teeth twice a day and have regular dental check-ups, but the benefits of this go far beyond keeping our teeth healthy. Brushing our teeth can also help keep our gums healthy and prevent periodontal disease. This starts as inflammation of the gums due to a bacterial film, and can spread to involve the bone.

Periodontal disease is associated with increased levels of inflammation, making it a risk factor for cardiac disease, dementia and diabetes. Healthy gums are a pale pink and should not bleed when you brush your teeth. As well as avoiding sugary drinks, it's also beneficial to visit your dentist regularly and ask them to show you how to brush your teeth and floss properly. Not only will this help you maintain a nice smile, it can also promote a healthy heart and brain, which are pretty great bonuses!

WHY ARE OLDER ADULTS MORE AT RISK FROM COVID-19?

They used to call pneumonia the old man's friend. I have looked after many people with pneumonia, seen them struggling to breathe and had to tell families that the one they love won't get better and I can tell you, pneumonia isn't friendly at all.

While the vast majority of people who develop COVID-19 have only mild symptoms and recover, around 5 per cent of people will have a more serious illness, and the most common organ to be severely affected is the lungs. At around day seven to ten of the illness, people can develop an inflammatory infiltrate in the air sacs of the lungs, meaning they fill with immune cells and fluid and it isn't possible to get enough oxygen.

While people in all age groups have died, overwhelmingly, the risk increases with age. In a study from Wuhan, the overall mortality for people aged over 80 was 14.8 per cent, almost double those aged seventy to seventy-nine. This is compared to 0.19 per cent for people aged twenty to twenty-nine.

COVID-19 is not the only disease that is more dangerous for older adults. Every year in flu season, even with a vaccine, older adults who are frail are more likely to die from the flu, or even to become very unwell with one of the regular cold viruses that would usually only cause a sniffle.

One of the key changes with age is that our immune systems become both more active and less efficient, which is called immunosenescence.

With age, comes a decrease in the ability to create anti-bodies, which are specific immune proteins that can target a particular microbe. This means that it is harder for older adults to control viral infections, because their immune systems don't have the same capability to produce anti-bodies. People who are older have faced far more infections than someone who is young, so with age we have less of a cell type called naïve T-cells, which are able to stimulate an antibody response to a new threat. This means that one of the key reasons older adults are more susceptible to COVID-19 is that they just aren't able to produce an effective antibody to control the disease.

While it would seem that the obvious solution is for the immune system to be as active as possible, unfettered immune activation can actually lead to damage of our own tissues.

One of the interesting things about COVID-19 is that people don't become very sick until day seven to ten of the disease. The timing makes it highly likely that an extremely strong immune response is actually causing some of the damage.

A key feature of immunosenescence is higher levels of inflammation. With age comes an accumulation of damaged cells, changes in cell signalling and changes in the gut microbiome that can all be drivers of inflammation. Combined with an ineffective antibody response, this loss of regulation of the immune response might also be contrib-uting to damage to the lungs and other organs.

One of the things that we don't know with COVID-19 is whether certain chronic diseases increase the risk of severe symptoms or if it is just that they are associated with age and frailty. Higher baseline levels of inflammation seem to play a role in the development of many chronic diseases including atherosclerosis and dementia. Inflammation is also associated with the development of frailty, which is characterised by having less reserve to cope with a stress like an infection.

Not all older adults will have the same susceptibility to this disease. While one person who is eighty might still be working, travelling and have a mean golf game, another might have serious health conditions and need assistance with activities of daily living. This can translate to a very different level of physical reserve to cope with a nasty virus that makes it hard to breathe.

These differences in health status are the result of a complex interplay of social, psychological, nutritional, genetic and medical factors that occur throughout life.

The regulation of our immune system and the role in fighting both infection and chronic disease is incredibly complex. A healthy immune system needs to be able to rapidly switch on to make a targeted antibody response and neutralise infection, and switch off to avoid damaging our own cells.

Since we know lifestyle steps including exercise, sleep and nutrition are excellent for staying well into older age and can impact immune function, this seems like a good place to start.

4

AGEING AND GUT HEALTH

If there is a healthy, established garden, it is harder for the weeds to grow.

Until the invention of the microscope a few hundred years ago, the world beyond the limits of human vision was invisible. Illness was thought to be due to bad air, miasmas or evil spirits. When microorganisms were first identified as the cause of disease, scientists learnt that improving hygiene and minimising exposure could help prevent disease outbreaks. This also led to the development of antibiotics, which made fatal infections treatable.

It is hard to quantify just how many lives have been saved by this understanding of microbes as a cause of disease. One of the first examples of germ theory being applied was in the UK. An English physician called John Snow didn't believe that cholera was caused by bad air; he thought it was caused by a small type of cell and was spread by people ingesting water that had been contaminated by faeces. Snow mapped the distribution of a cholera outbreak in London in 1854 and traced it back to a water pump, which was contaminated from a nearby cesspool. By convincing the water authorities to disable the pump, he ended the cholera outbreak.

Germ theory helped drive one of the most lifesaving public health developments of the 1800s: a sewage system.

It is only very recently that we have started to recognise that many microbes are actually very helpful, and are not just sources of disease. These bacteria, viruses and yeasts form part of a complex ecosystem called the microbiome. This covers every part of your body that is exposed to the outside world, including the skin, the vagina, the airways and the digestive tract. The microbiome in your mouth is populated by very different species to the one in your bowel. Even different parts of your skin will each have their own microbiome: as you can appreciate, the conditions in your armpit are quite different to those on your face.

Our gut microbiome

In the simplest terms, the gut is a continuous tube from the mouth to the anus. However, every section has a specialised role and a specialised microbiome. In our mouth, food is chewed and mixed with saliva to mechanically break it down and start the digestive process. Once we swallow a mouthful of food, our oesophagus propels it to our stomach with a wave-like contraction. After it enters the acidic environment of the stomach, a one-way valve is supposed to stop it from going back where it came from, although anyone who has had reflux will know this doesn't always work. After being mushed around in the stomach for a while, the food passes to the small intestine, where it is mixed with more digestive enzymes to break it into fats, carbohydrates and proteins so it can be absorbed by the cells there. The remnants then pass into the large intestine, which starts in your lower right abdomen, travels up towards your liver, takes a left turn past your spleen, then heads down towards the exit.

How does your garden grow?

Each individual's gut microbiome is so specific that some people have suggested it could be used in forensics, like a fingerprint.

When we are born, we are 'seeded' with bacteria, which is either from the vagina or from the skin, for those born by caesarean. Breastmilk also contains milk oligosaccharides, which are complex sugars that promote the growth of certain types of bacteria. There are other influences on the infant's microbiome, including starting solid foods, interacting with pets, needing antibiotics for illness, not to mention the broad range of objects that all babies try to put in their mouths as part of their sensory development. (I'm sure that the day my toddler ate mud from a cow paddock he increased his microbiome markedly!)

While the gut microbiome stabilises at around age three, environmental factors still have a big influence. Not surprisingly, the foods you eat will affect which species of bacteria predominate. Exercise can also change the balance of bacterial species in the gut microbiome, although most of the research supporting this is in mice. People who smoke tend to have lower levels of microbial diversity. Commonly used medications can also alter the microbiome. Although we know that these things affect our microbiome, we still don't know if the effect is good or bad.

The large intestine is the site of the largest and most diverse collection of microbes in our body. These bacteria break down fibre (the part of plant cells that we are not able to digest with our own enzymes), creating short-chain fatty acids (SCFAs) as by-products. The three main SCFAs are acetate, propionate and butyrate. They not only provide food for our intestinal cells, keeping our gut wall healthy, they also have a role in metabolism, immune function and many other bodily processes.

COULD GUT BUGS PLAY A ROLE IN OBESITY?

The gut microbiome may play a direct causal role in obesity. This has been well studied in mice, including breeding mice that are microbe-free, then transplanting gut microbes from both lean and obese mice. The mice that received these transplants then developed body types that were consistent with the donor mice. Not surprisingly, this hasn't been as well studied in humans, but one very interesting study took men with impaired sensitivity to insulin, cleaned out their small intestines, then added in either their own microbes again or donor microbes from people who were lean. In the men who received the donor microbes, their sensitivity to insulin actually improved. This is very early data, and a long way from being a clinical treatment, but offers an intriguing insight into our relationship with our microbes.

In a fascinating study led by Professor Gary Frost at Imperial College London, researchers recruited 60 people to examine the effect of a propionate supplement on appetite and weight gain. Propionate is one of the SCFAs produced by gut microbes when they digest fibre, and the researchers wanted to work out its impact on appetite. The subjects were randomly assigned to receive either the supplement or a placebo. The results showed that people on the supplement were less likely to gain weight and had lower levels of fat tissue after the trial. Although the people who were taking the supplement did not report lower appetite, they actually ate smaller meals. When the researchers looked at intestinal cells in the laboratory, they found a probable reason for this. Putting propionate in the test tube with the intestinal cells caused them to make hormones called peptide YY (PYY) and glucagon-like peptide-1, which are known to suppress appetite. Although blood tests revealed that the levels of these hormones weren't measurably higher, there still seemed to be some sort of appetite suppression from the propionate. Perhaps for us to feel full, our microbes need their hunger sated too. This might explain why fibre can help regulate appetite.

The gut and the immune system

I'm sure almost everyone reading this has had food poisoning at some time, and vividly recalls how horrible it is. Some food- and water-borne bacteria and viruses can be incredibly serious. Cholera is a bacterium that is found in contaminated water supplies and has caused fatal outbreaks. Hepatitis A is a virus that can come from contaminated food and causes acute inflammation of the liver, and salmonella typhi (typhoid) is a virus that can cause blood infections (sepsis). These and other pathogens (such as worms and other parasites) are why most of the body's immune cells are found in the gut.

The microbiome has been with us since long before we were human – the earliest single-celled organisms probably had their own interactions with microbes. At the same time, there has always been an ongoing need to balance these microbes so that we can benefit from them and not become overwhelmed (and so they, in turn, do not lose their host). This means that our immune systems have had to learn to tolerate these commensal bacteria. For example, when the intestinal cells detect butyrate, one of the SCFAs, it leads to the release of the cytokine IL-18, which in turn activates t-regulatory cells, putting the brakes on the immune system.

The good bacteria that live in our gut can play a key role in keeping the bad guys from getting a look-in. If there is a healthy, established garden, it is harder for the weeds to grow.

SCFAs AND GUT WALL INTEGRITY

In recent years, there has been a lot of discussion around the idea of 'leaky gut syndrome'. Although this is a controversial term in medical circles, it refers to an important concept. A more scientific term is 'altered intestinal permeability'. The cells in the small and large intestine have dual roles: they need to let nutrients in while also protecting the inside of the body from the many potentially problematic substances that pass through the gut. This is maintained by the tight connections between the gut cells and a layer of mucous on the surface of the intestines.

The problematic substances include lipopolysaccharides, bacterial products that induce inflammation. In animal models, these have been linked to the development of atherosclerosis, neuroinflammation and chronic disease.

While increased intestinal permeability has been linked to many conditions, including food allergy, cirrhosis and Parkinson's disease, there is still no definitive proof. There is no test to medically diagnose leaky gut, and we don't have specific treatments for it. There is also no evidence that making the gut less leaky will actually have health benefits.

One way to optimise gut health is to eat lots of fibre. While many of the bacteria in our gut prefer to 'eat' fibre, if there isn't enough fibre they will swap to the protective mucous. Providing your microbes a good supply of fibre will also give them the right substrate to produce short-chain fatty acids which can actually stimulate gut cells in a way that enhances the mucous barrier.

The gut and the brain

Amazingly, the gut is sometimes called the second brain because it actually contains as many neurons as the brain of a cat. This is the enteric nervous system, which is responsible for coordinating our digestion. We want our food to proceed in an orderly fashion from our mouth to our anus, allowing the right amount of time in the stomach, small intestine and large intestine so that all of the nutrients are extracted. Your second brain won't be writing the next great literary masterpiece, but it does communicate with your 'main' brain via the vagus nerve to feed back critical information about body function.

The vagus nerve extends from the brain stem (the part of the brain at the top of the spinal cord) to the digestive system, and also has fibres that go to the heart, the diaphragm and the lungs. The brain stem is the 'survival' part of our brains; it controls breathing, blood pressure, heart rate, alertness and arousal. The vagus nerve wanders through the body, with connections to the throat to control swallowing and speaking, the heart to control heart rate, and the intestines to control the rate of muscle contraction and secretion of digestive fluids. It is also responsible for sneezing, coughing and vomiting.

Around 80–90 per cent of the fibres in the vagus nerve carry sensory information from the gut back to the brain. This is one of the ways that our appetite is regulated; the vagus nerve tells the brain that the stomach and intestines have been stretched. The vagus nerve also has connections to parts of the brain controlled in emotional regulation. It is not clear whether this directly influences mood or behaviour (maybe this explains why we get hangry!), but the therapeutic potential is being explored.

Our microbes can talk to our brains

The messages the vagus nerve carries back to our brain are also influenced by our microbes. Our microbes need us to stay alive in order to maintain their own habitat. Just as in a forest with plants competing for sunlight, there are many different species of microorganisms, and they take active steps to make their homes comfortable and to compete with other species. Many symbionts, aka friendly bacteria, actually make their own neurotransmitters. These might act to alter the local environment to make it more favourable for themselves, and may even influence behaviour.

Some research has shown a link between the microbiome and depression. A 2016 study published in the *Journal of Psychiatric Research* showed that people with depression had decreased diversity in their microbiome. The researchers took this one step further and transplanted faecal samples from depressed people into rats. The rats subsequently displayed behavioural changes consistent with rat depression. Obviously humans have far more complex behavioural patterns than rats, so we can't directly extrapolate from this study, but it adds to the growing evidence that a healthy microbiome might be good for your mental health.

These studies are compelling, but it is impossible to know which parts of the microbiome are actually clinically significant. A 2019 study published in *Nature Microbiology* helps to answer this question. The study looked at two cohorts, one in Belgium and another in the Netherlands, and measured quality of life and the faecal microbiome. The researchers consistently found that in people with lower quality of life, two species of bacteria were depleted: Faecalibacterium and Coprococcus. It is possible that these bacteria were consistently associated with higher quality of life indicators because they produce the SCFA butyrate. Despite being the least abundant SCFA, butyrate is the major nutrition source for the cells lining the colon. It also has anti-inflammatory effects, and can repair and enhance the barrier function of intestinal cells. This improvement in gut health by decreasing inflammation and providing protection from bacterial lipopolysaccharides, as well as the influence on vagal nerve function, might explain why a healthy microbiome enhances mood.

How our digestion changes with ageing

There are age-associated changes in the gut and digestion. The first area we may notice change is in the mouth. Periodontal disease is an important risk factor for the development of many conditions, including diabetes, dementia and frailty. This is likely to be because poor dental health and inflamed gums can lead to increased exposure to bacteria, which drives further inflammation.

As we age, the peristaltic contractions that push food through the gut can become less coordinated, increasing the time it takes for food to get through the digestive system. At the most severe, this can lead to a condition called nutcracker oesophagus, where the oesophagus spasms so badly that no food can get down at all. It also may explain why constipation increases with age.

In older age a less diverse gut microbiome has been linked with frailty. In one study, frail older adults who lived in residential care had fewer bacterial species than a group of matched controls who lived in the community. This may be related to their diet or the medications they require – all of which may impact the microbiome.

Other studies have looked at the microbiome in centenarians, who have obviously cracked the code to achieving a very long life. Even within this group, there doesn't seem to be one bacterial species that holds the key to longevity. Instead, like many natural ecosystems, a greater variety of species indicates health. However, even though there is an association between a higher level of diversity in the microbiome and staying healthy into old age, this does not prove causation. It is possible that the changes of inflammaging drive changes in the microbiome, rather than the other way around. To discern which comes first, researchers would need to follow people for a longer period of time to see if changes in the microbiome preceded frailty or vice versa. Only then could we start to explore whether treating the gut microbiome might improve physical functioning as we age.

FAECAL MICROBIOTA TRANSPLANT (FMT)

The bacteria *Clostridioides difficile* (C. diff) got its name because it was originally very difficult to culture, and it has since lived up to its name because it can be so difficult to treat. C. diff causes diarrhoea and inflammation in the colon. It is treated by antibiotics, but can be very hard to eradicate. The most common risk factor for C. diff is recent treatment with antibiotics, followed by age. I have had patients who would need course after course of antibiotics, becoming weaker and weaker after each flare-up. Sometimes C. diff could cause such severe inflammation in the large intestine that the sufferer required emergency surgery to remove part of the bowel.

In recent years, a new treatment has revolutionised the treatment of recurrent C. diff infection: faecal transplant. In the small proportion of patients who do not respond to antibiotics, faeces is taken from a healthy donor, usually a relative, blended to a liquid and introduced via a colonoscopy.

Giving their microbiome a boost of healthy bacteria cures around 70–90 per cent of patients who have not responded to antibiotics. When the colon is repopulated by a 'normal' microbiome, the conditions are no longer so favourable for C. diff, and it loses its foothold.

So, should you be finding a fit, young person and asking them for some poo? At this stage the answer is a firm no. We just don't know enough about what makes a good microbiota. There are also potential harms involved, such as acquiring an infection or even perforating your bowel. Definitely not something you should try at home!

Probiotics or prebiotics for a healthy microbiome?

Probiotic foods are those that contain living bacteria and other organisms. Prebiotic foods are those that feed our gut microbiome, such as those high in fibre.

One question I am frequently asked is: 'Should I take probiotic supplements?' These are capsules containing friendly bacteria that are marketed as easy ways to replenish your gut microbiome. While the potential therapeutic applications of this are fascinating, so far the research is far from convincing. For a probiotic capsule to cause a change in microbial make-up, they would not only need to be introduced in a viable state in high numbers, they'd also have to survive the trip through stomach acid and other digestive hurdles, and then successfully compete with resident microbiota for nutritional resources to thrive.

There is some evidence that probiotics can shorten the duration of infectious diarrhoea in children, and that they may help relieve constipation in older adults. There is not yet any evidence that they have a role in chronic disease, but time and further studies will help answer this question.

Uncooked, fermented foods are another way to introduce more species of bacteria to your gut. Humans are known to have used fermentation to preserve foods since Neolithic times (mostly wine, beer and bread made with yeasts). Later, fermentation (using bacteria and moulds) was used to make cheese, yoghurt and other milk products, as well as pickled vegetables such as sauerkraut and kimchi, and drinks such as kombucha.

Studies of faecal samples from people who have eaten fermented foods have shown that it is possible for some of the friendly bacteria (such as Lactobacillus) to survive the journey to the large intestine. There is also some evidence that eating yoghurt may reduce symptoms of irritable bowel disease. Researchers have also found that people who eat lots of fermented foods such as kimchi, tempeh (fermented soybeans), miso and yoghurt have a lower risk of developing type 2 diabetes.

It's not clear if the benefit of fermented foods is just from the boosted microbial population. The bacteria and yeasts that partly break down the food also unlock many of its nutrients, which we would otherwise not be able to access. Bread is an excellent example of this. Traditional sourdough bread-making involves wholegrain flour and water that is left to its own devices in a warm place, allowing the natural microbes (yeast and lactobacilli) to break down the flour. The dough is left to 'prove' for anywhere from 8 to 24 hours.

In 1961 the Chorleywood process was developed, which cut the proving time to about an hour and enabled bread to be produced on a mass scale, but this means there isn't time for the microbes to ferment the flour. Since the partial digestion of the flour by the microorganisms increases the availability of nutrients, including amino acids and B-vitamins, this means that while modern, industrial bread-making is efficient, it results in a far less nutritious product. We do know that people who follow a traditional lifestyle and eat around 100 grams of fibre a day have far higher levels of diversity in their poop than those of us living in Western societies. The best thing you can do for your microbiome is to eat a wide variety of plant foods in their natural state, including root veggies, leafy greens, salad veggies, fruit, nuts, seeds and wholegrains. This will encourage a diverse and healthy community in your gut.

DON'T BOTHER WITH POO ANALYSIS (YET)

At the moment, it is possible to send your poo away to be analysed, even down to the genes present in your microbiome. Beyond satisfying your curiosity, I do not recommend this because there is still so much we don't know about the microbiota. The bacteria that we have identified and know more about are the ones that are easiest to grow. Imagine going to the deepest depths of the ocean and catching a fish; this fish cannot be kept alive in the air. Many bacteria are similar: they require specific conditions to grow, so we still can't actually grow most bacteria in the laboratory. When the DNA of the microbiome is analysed, it is full of species that aren't even known to science. This means that the secret to improving your health is still going to be to eat your veggies.

5

AGEING, STRESS AND MENTAL HEALTH

Our minds are an incredibly powerful tool to improve longevity.

One of the most striking things I have learned from working with older adults is how resilient people can be. It is a rare life that is not marked by hardship and loss in some way. Whether it is the death of a loved one, a change in financial circumstances or a health scare, people have an incredible capacity to take on stress and keep living.

Put simply, stress is the mind and body's reaction to anything that we perceive as a threat. Short, sharp bursts of stress, like a ride on a roller-coaster or preparing for an exam, are probably good for us. It is when stress is chronic, severe and feels beyond our control that it is linked with health problems.

Severe stressful life events, such as a sudden bereavement, are not good for us, and are particularly bad for our hearts. Researchers consistently report a spike in sudden cardiac-related deaths following a natural disaster. Even just a few weeks of low-level stress puts a strain on our bodies and minds through changes in our neuro-hormonal system. The environment we live in can affect our very cells, right down to the rate of ageing. This is why chronic stress is recognised as a risk factor for heart disease.

MARIA'S STORY

Maria came to see me because she wasn't sleeping.

When I probed a little further, there was more behind this. She couldn't sleep because it was coming up to the one-year anniversary of her daughter's death. Maria's beloved middle daughter had died unexpectedly, and she was finding it incredibly hard to go on living. Her other children wanted to find ways to help her to recover, but on speaking to Maria, I don't think this is what she wanted. Maria's grief was deep, acute and profound. It had changed everything about her and she couldn't see a way to engage with life. At night all she could think about at night was that she would never see her daughter again.

We often talk about people 'getting over' trauma, resolving and moving on.

I think that it is important to acknowledge that we can't resolve all losses. Certain losses remain breathtakingly sharp, no matter how distant. I think that it can be important to sit with someone and to respect their deep sadness. I have met many people who have lost a child and no matter how long ago it happened, the grief never goes, and nor should we expect it to.

The biology of stress

Last night I was watching the finale of a thrilling TV series. I was literally sitting on the edge of my seat, muscles tensed, heart pounding. Even though the conscious part of my brain knew that the actors were not really in danger, the more primitive part of my brain was responding to a perceived threat in the only way it knew how: by sending signals to prepare me to face it or run.

When we see, hear or smell something that indicates a threat, we have the fight or flight response, preparing us to either go into battle or run away. Our pupils dilate to improve our vision, our heart beats faster to deliver more oxygen to our muscles and brain, and our liver releases glucose for an instant energy hit.

This response makes sense in an evolutionary context, since for most of our history we were hunter-gatherers, and physical threats, such as attacks from predators or rivals, were a big concern. However, this response is not so useful if we're sitting on the couch watching a gripping murder mystery, or sitting at our desk after a stressful phone call. It is especially damaging when we experience it many times a day, day after day.

Our brain has two ways of getting the body ready for a physical confrontation: via the sympathetic nervous system (SNS) and the hypothalamic-pituitary-adrenal (HPA) axis.

The sympathetic nervous system (SNS)

Along with the parasympathetic nervous system and the enteric nervous system, the SNS is the third component of the autonomic nervous system. The sympathetic nervous system acts in the opposite way to the parasympathetic nervous system. Where the parasympathetic nervous system is in charge when we are resting and digesting, the SNS kicks in when it is time for physical action.

The SNS connects our brain to our heart, lungs, liver and other organs through our spinal nerves. This means that when we see, hear or smell a threat, our brain can rapidly send a signal via these nerves to prepare us to face danger by increasing our heart rate, boosting blood flow to our muscles, dilating our pupils etc. It also acts to decrease blood supply to the gut. This gets us ready for strenuous physical activity. The SNS also connects to the adrenal medulla, the inner section of the adrenal glands, which sit on top of the kidneys and release adrenaline into the bloodstream. This circulating adrenaline can make blood vessels constrict, which, in turn, can raise blood pressure. This is why some people get 'white coat hypertension', where they get so nervous about having their blood pressure checked that their blood pressure actually goes up.

Cortisol and the HPA axis

HPA stands for hypothalamic-pituitary-adrenal and describes the cascade of signals our brains use to regulate cortisol release. Our nervous system is one mechanism for body-wide communication; the other is hormones. Nerves transmit electrical signals extremely rapidly to and from the brain, where hormones are released into the blood by endocrine glands, like the pancreas and thyroid.

Cortisol is a hormone essential to many bodily processes, including blood sugar regulation, blood pressure control and immune function. In a rare disorder where people can't make cortisol, they actually die without treatment.

When we see or hear a threat, corticotropin-releasing factor (CRF) is released from the hypothalamus, a structure in the brain, which stimulates the secretion of adrenocorticotropin (ACTH) from the pituitary gland, which is right next to the hypothalamus.

ACTH in turn stimulates the synthesis and release of cortisol from the adrenal glands, which sit just on top of our kidneys.

Cortisol levels have a diurnal variation: there is a spike in cortisol every morning at around the time we wake up, then levels fall through the day. Cortisol impacts the gene expression of more than two hundred genes and we still have more to learn about its actions.

One of the big differences between the sympathetic nervous system and the HPA axis is the time they take to turn on and off. The SNS turns on and off almost instantaneously; the HPA axis takes around fifteen minutes to get going and can take hours to wear off.

If you imagine a soldier going into battle, a spike of cortisol is very useful. Having a higher level of this hormone in the blood will improve physical performance and increase the risk of surviving an injury. Similarly to the SNS, cortisol increases blood pressure and blood clotting, which is very useful for a sword injury. It also increases glucose levels in the blood, which means there is ready energy available for active muscles. Cortisol actually enhances memory, which might be useful for avoiding future threats. Short bursts of cortisol also increase levels of inflammation, which is useful if you are expecting an injury – inflammation is part of the healing process.

Normally, once the hypothalamus detects that cortisol has been released, it stops producing CRF so we don't keep making more cortisol. However, this negative feedback loop can be disrupted in some people, especially those exposed to chronically high levels of stress. People who are stressed continue to secrete cortisol, even when levels are already high. When cortisol release stays high for a prolonged time, it has wide-ranging effects, as we will see in the next section.

The metabolic effects of chronic stress

Higher blood pressure, increased blood glucose and a hyper-alert brain are all very helpful if you are able to physically deal with stress. These changes that cortisol induces are very useful when you are about to have a burst of physical activity, but if they are chronic and related to a tight work deadline that involves sitting for hours at your computer, they are not so functional. Over the longer term, high levels of blood glucose and blood pressure have negative effects on many body systems.

Over years, high blood pressure can change the structure of arteries and this can contribute to atherosclerosis. Similarly, long-term elevation of blood glucose due to cortisol may be a mechanism linking psychosocial stress and diabetes. Over the long-term, cortisol also has an impact on body composition. Cortisol can lead to increased abdominal fat and lower muscle and bone mass.

The Whitehall Study, which follows a group of people, has been running in the UK for decades. One of the things researchers have looked at is the relationship between cortisol levels and chronic disease. In one part of the study, salivary cortisol was measured many times over a single day. The researcher found that a flat pattern of cortisol release – meaning that levels weren't falling as the day went on – was associated with diabetes. Two years later, the researchers went back and looked at the people with a 'flat' pattern of cortisol release who didn't have diabetes. At follow-up, these people were slightly more likely to have a new diagnosis of diabetes or impaired glucose tolerance, which is a precursor to diabetes. In the short term, cortisol can suppress (down-regulate) the immune system, but if there is long-term elevation of cortisol, its regulatory effects are lost, and the immune system can become overactive. As we saw earlier, this may contribute to elevated systemic inflammation. This is another mechanism that links chronic levels of stress with inflammation, ageing and disease.

The relationship between cortisol, inflammation and disease is complex. Although higher cortisol levels are associated with obesity, we're not sure which way the relationship runs: it could be that stress and cortisol drive obesity, but it could also be the other way around. It is also possible that a higher level of baseline inflammation can drive higher cortisol levels and obesity.

Since cortisol affects the function of so many genes, it is not surprising that changes in its patterns of secretion could also alter cellular ageing. Cortisol increases the secretion of IGF-1, which may push our cells away from repair pathways, further increasing rates of ageing. There is an association between high levels of self-reported stress and shorter telomeres, although the effect is small.

Overall, one bad day isn't going to have a long-term effect on health, but years of bad days might. This means that one of the unfair things in life is that those who are already doing it tough also pay the price of poorer health.

POVERTY AND HEALTH

When I went from working in one of the wealthiest parts of Melbourne to one of the poorest, the average age of my patients dropped by ten years. Quite simply, their lives had been so much harder that they were sick at a younger age.

My clinical experience is confirmed by research from the UK, which showed that people with an income in the lowest tertile have a health status equivalent to those ten years older in the highest tertile. The city of Glasgow provides another staggering example: in the poorest part of the city, life expectancy for men is 54, compared to 82 in the wealthiest parts. This gap was created after the collapse of the coal industry saw massive unemployment and the breakdown of social structures.

Being poor is stressful. There is the worry of paying the rent, job uncertainty and how to afford food. It is socially isolating. It can also mean living in a less desirable part of a city, with little access to open spaces that are safe and pleasant to walk in. For someone whose mind is fully occupied by all these worries, there is no space to plan health strategies for the future: surviving today is enough.

The impact of socio-economic factors on physical health is real and it's not just from associations with smoking, drug use and poorer access to nutritious food. It has measurable effects on hormone levels and inflammation.

As a clinician, I feel particularly helpless seeing people with chronic health conditions and knowing that some of the risk for this is from the hard lives they have been born into. It feels incredibly trite to suggest relaxation techniques to people who are struggling to feed themselves and their families. I feel like the best I can offer is to listen and learn. This is also why I feel very strongly that, as a society, we need to care about other people and to have a focus on fairness and equality.

There are factors that are within our control, but we also need public health support to put wellbeing within everyone's reach.

Chronic stress and mental health

We all have times when we feel sad or anxious, and these are often tied to stressful life changes, such as loss of work, conflict with colleagues, relationship break-ups, illness in the family or the death of someone we love. While it is normal to have these feelings at times, not surprisingly, chronic stress is a risk factor for developing depression or anxiety.

In countries like the US, UK and Australia, around 30 per cent of the population experiences anxiety or depression at some time in their lives, and these conditions are more prevalent in women. Although many older adults experience loss and grief, rates of depression actually decrease in older age, although for people managing chronic disease, such as heart disease or diabetes, depression is markedly increased.

While some people will only experience one episode of depression, over the years around half will have another occurrence. Major depression is usually diagnosed after someone experiences more than two weeks of symptoms that interfere with their ability to do normal daily tasks. These symptoms include: a persistent low mood; feelings of worthlessness; lack of interest and enjoyment in usual activities; disturbed sleep (insomnia or hypersomnia) and changes in appetite.

Anxiety disorders include obsessive compulsive disorder, panic disorder, social anxiety disorder and generalised anxiety disorder, all of which cause distress and impair function.

Anxiety and depression frequently overlap, and many people will have symptoms of both.

While we often think of the brain and body as being separate, we need to remember that the brain is also made of cells, which need a good blood supply to bring nutrients and oxygen at all times. Although we are capable of incredibly complex thoughts, we are still just animals that are very much beholden to our physical needs. The day I am writing this is extremely hot, which makes me want to go into the shade. I feel a dry sensation in my mouth and

I seek water; I don't feel like moving much. The sensations in our body, our physical needs, drive many of our everyday decisions.

Although psychiatry is a separate medical specialty, the reality is that our physical and mental states are not separate. This has been particularly well studied in heart disease, where we know that people who have depression are at a higher risk of heart attack. We also know that heart attacks are a risk for depression, and that in people who are depressed after a heart attack, the risk of dying is four times higher.

Mental and physical health have a bidirectional relationship. This enhances our understanding of disease, provides potential therapies and highlights the need for holistic care.

There is evidence that inflammation itself may be a contributing factor to depression. For example, we know that in patients with hepatitis C who are treated with the drug interferon-alpha, about half will develop depression. This is because interferon-alpha increases immune system activation. Indeed, multiple population studies have found that, on average, people with depression have higher levels of inflammation. Fascinatingly, data from the Whitehall Study showed that people who had higher levels of inflammation at baseline were more likely to have developed symptoms of depression when they were followed up years later.

Although inflammation has been associated with depression in many studies, it is worth remembering that in many cases, inflammation alone is not enough. Depression and anxiety are the result of a complex interplay between genetic, environmental, social and physical factors. Not all people treated with the immune-inducing drug interferon-alpha will experience depression, and not all people with depression will have raised levels of inflammation. Human health, particularly mental health, is complex, and sometimes different processes can lead to the same symptoms.

If anyone reading this is worried that they may have symptoms of anxiety or depression, I urge you to make an appointment to see your family doctor as soon as possible. Some people will need treatment with medications that can, at times, be lifesaving. There are also evidence-based lifestyle strategies that can help to manage these conditions. Seeking help is a brave and positive first step.

HEATHER'S STORY

Heather's horror year started when her father was found walking along a highway headed to the workplace he had retired from many years prior. Heather had recognised that her father's dementia had been worsening over the previous few years, and despite living over an hour away from him, regularly visited to provide practical support. When Heather got the call that her father had been found by someone he knew walking along a highway to the workplace he had retired from ten years earlier, she and her siblings knew that it was time for him to move into residential care. Heather's dad was very upset because he could not understand why he needed to leave his home. As a result, Heather was left with incredible guilt, as well as the practicalities of sorting through his house. Shortly afterwards Heather's aunt died, and again it fell to her to manage all the administration that comes with end of life. Then, unbelievably, Heather's husband was diagnosed with throat cancer. During his treatment she had to help him three times a day with his nasogastric feeds.

To say Heather was stressed is an understatement, but she was able to draw on both internal and external reserves. Heather found that the support of her friends was crucial, as well as that of her children, but she also had her own technique: on her regular long drives she would scream and yell about how unfair everything was. This emotional release made her feel better. Importantly, she didn't dwell on the anger, but rather focused on doing what needed to be done.

How to buffer stress

I don't want anyone reading this to start feeling bad about being stressed – it's a normal part of life. Even small things like misplacing your keys or getting caught in a traffic jam can trigger the neuro-hormonal response I described earlier.

Fortunately, there are some things we can change in life to decrease our stress levels, such as prioritising what is important to us and saying no to extra commitments that would be a drain on our emotional energy. However, even if we take steps to remove avoidable stressors, not everything is under our control. This is why it is important to use strategies to modulate our stress response.

Abdominal breathing

When people are anxious, breathing can become shallow and rapid. Focused and controlled breathing is part of many ancient practices, such as yoga, tai chi and meditation. Utilising some of these techniques can be a way to manage symptoms of anxiety.

Sometimes called diaphragmatic breathing, this is a technique you can use to help your mind and body relax. These steps are modified from yoga:

1. Place your palms on your abdomen with your fingertips just touching.

2. Inhale deeply into your abdomen by 'pushing out' your belly (you'll know you're doing it well if your fingers move slightly apart).
3. Exhale slowly and fully.
4. Keeping your hands on your abdomen, inhale deeply for four counts, hold for four counts and then exhale for four counts.

If you keep this up, you may actually feel your heart rate begin to slow. The reason this works is still not completely understood. It may relate to the vagus nerve's role in feeding back information about the body to the mind; when your breathing slows, your brain gets the idea that everything is okay and you don't need to be in a state of high alert. If practised regularly, this may have an impact on cortisol levels (although the study that showed this was small, with some methodological issues).

Regardless, it is a useful tool to have in your kit when life gets tricky!

Mindfulness

Mindfulness is non-judgemental, present-focused attention. It is training the mind to stay where we are – not worrying about the past or planning the future, just noticing and accepting what is happening in the moment. Of course, this takes practice. Most of us (including me) are not able to sit still and peacefully observe our thoughts (I generally end up making a mental to-do list!). Fortunately, there are other ways to help bring our minds back to the present moment, and these often involve doing things we love, such as cooking, gardening, walking, dancing, swimming, yoga or painting. Doing any activity where you can find a sense of flow or deep concentration can be mentally refreshing and may have the same benefits as mindfulness.

Exercise and heat

In the Royal Australian and New Zealand College of Psychiatrists, exercise is a recommended treatment (in conjunction with other therapies) for mild to moderate depression. This is because both aerobic and resistance training have been shown to decrease symptoms of depression. This is likely due to multiple factors. Exercise has complex effects on the immune system. When we exercise, our muscles release the inflammatory cytokine IL-6. This is partly because exercise can cause small amounts of muscle damage that the body needs to repair. Interestingly in the context of everything else going on in the body when we exercise, this cytokine also has an anti-inflammatory effect; some researchers think this might explain why exercise can decrease inflammation and improve mood. When we exercise more of our blood also travels to the brain, and this can change patterns of neurotransmitters.

Another evolving treatment for depression is sauna use. In a well-designed randomised controlled trial, researchers recruited people with depression and randomly assigned half to heat and half to a sham heat box. The intervention group were 'cooked' until their internal temperature was 38 degrees Celsius. After a single treatment, at six weeks the intervention group had a lower depression score. Sauna use seems to activate many of the same pathways as exercise. Although this is only a small trial, and to my knowledge it hasn't been repeated, it is still promising as a novel therapy for depression.

ALCOHOL AND MENTAL HEALTH

In our society it's not always acceptable to talk about your problems, but drinking alcohol to try to forget them is. While alcohol can be extremely enjoyable, if you are drinking to treat symptoms of anxiety or depression, it might be a good idea to talk to your doctor about taking a break. Here's why.

A glass of wine can seem like a great way to relax after a difficult day, but it can actually make anxiety worse. As anyone who has felt a little tipsy after a glass of wine would attest, alcohol can freely cross the blood–brain barrier and wreak havoc in the brain, where it can have complex effects. It makes people less inhibited, but it is also a sedative, which is why people fall asleep after too many drinks. This complex action is because alcohol acts on multiple neurotransmitters, including serotonin, GABA and glutamate. People who drink alcohol regularly can experience changes in expression of receptors for some of these neurotransmitters, which could explain why habitual drinkers can tolerate higher levels of alcohol intake. Alcohol also activates our reward pathway, and this combination of tolerance and reward is why alcohol is addictive. For people who are already feeling depressed or anxious, these changes in the expression of neurotransmitters will amplify those feelings.

Stress can also be great

During my years training as a specialist physician, every time I would move up to a new level of responsibility it was an additional layer of stress. This was combined with studying for extremely challenging exams. Being on this steep learning curve was extremely challenging and of course stressful, but it was also incredible to reflect on my own achievements and growth.

Working towards an important goal is stressful, but it can also be an extremely positive part of life. This phenomenon is called stress-related growth, where the experience can foster new learning and add meaning to life.

One of the most important strategies for stress is to have a positive mindset, to recognise that stress can be a good thing because it means that you are challenging yourself. Emotional support, regular exercise and adequate sleep are all key strategies to manage stress to get the most out of life.

6

THE MALE–FEMALE
LONGEVITY PARADOX

Women live longer than men, but in poorer health.

Walking through the dining room at a residential aged care facility at lunch time, I see tables full of women all eating and chatting happily, with only the occasional man. One reason for this is that in every country of the world women have a longer life expectancy than men. Another is that although women live longer, we are also more likely to have chronic health conditions and to need help with essential activities of daily living in older age.

This phenomenon is called the male–female health survival paradox: women live longer than men, but in poorer health. UN data from 2013 showed that 85 men per 100 women were aged 60 years or over, and 61 men per 100 women were aged 80 years or over. In 2016 worldwide life expectancy was 67 years for males and 71.1 years for females, although this varies significantly by country. This increased life expectancy for women has been seen as far back as there are records of births and deaths. Even in past centuries when many women did not survive childbirth, women still had a longer average life expectancy.

The almost universal aspect of this increased life expectancy highlights that there is a significant biological component. There is something about being a woman that increases the chance of surviving, ranging from a decreased susceptibility to infection to much later presentations of cardiac disease.

THE RUSSIAN STORY

Russia has the biggest male–female gap in life expectancy in the world, at a huge 11.3 years. To make sense of this, it is important to understand some of Russia's recent social history and current gender norms.

Russia had a tumultuous last century, with significant social upheaval. World War I was particularly brutal, with peasants essentially used as cannon fodder on the Western Front to hold off Germany. This, combined with gross inequality, lead to the Bolshevik revolution in 1917, when Tsar Alexander and his family were overthrown by Lenin and his Communist comrades, who then struggled to rule the shattered country. World War II was a time of monumental savagery for Russians. The Germans marched through the countryside stealing and destroying food supplies. This, combined with military casualties, led to the death of around 20 million people. Yet Russia's trauma did not end after the war. Stalin's reign of terror saw 750,000 people sent to the Gulags in Siberia, where most died in the terrible conditions or were executed.

Although standards of living and education progressively improved in the decades that followed, the experiences of war had significant repercussions for the men of subsequent generations. In a culture where being masculine means being stoic and not admitting to emotional distress, Russian men have few socially acceptable coping strategies – except drinking. Around 25 per cent of Russian men drink alcohol more than twice a week, compared to just 3.9 per cent of women. A study of three Siberian towns in the 1990s found that around 52 per cent of deaths of men and women aged 15–52 were due to excess alcohol. Russian men are also more likely to smoke, which is another likely contributor to higher rates of cancer and cardiovascular disease.

The Russian version of masculinity, the stoic man who drinks away his pain, is deadly.

Genetic influences

Slightly more boys are born than girls, but from birth onwards, males have a higher rate of mortality. One of the survival advantages that women have is two X chromosomes. Each cell of our body (other than a sperm or ova) has 23 pairs of chromosomes, which are strands of DNA. Each chromosome in a pair has the same genes in the same locations, although the exact instructions for each gene may differ: one chromosome may contain a gene that encodes a protein that will lead to blue eyes, while the corresponding gene in the other chromosome encodes a protein that will result in brown eyes. Both genes are fully functional, but will lead to a different appearance. An advantage of the two chromosomes is that one can provide a 'backup' copy of a defective gene.

Fertilisation takes place when a sperm meets an ova. Each sperm and ova has 23 unpaired chromosomes. The ova, from the woman, contains an X chromosome and the sperm, from the man, can have either an X or a Y chromosome, so the type of sperm that fertilises the ova will determine the biological sex of the embryo. There are around 3000 to 5000 genes on the X chromosome, including genes involved in immune function, blood clotting, muscle structure and the ability to see colour. The Y chromosome is visibly much smaller than the X chromosome, and contains around 200 genes. This means that many of the genes that are on the X chromosome are not contained on the Y chromosome, which is why some genetic conditions such as colour blindness and Duchenne muscular dystrophy are seen almost exclusively in men: they inherit the defective gene from their mother, who is not affected because she has a functioning copy on her other X chromosome.

When there are two active copies of chromosomes, usually one copy of each gene will be randomly turned off during development. For men, their one X chromosome will always be turned on, but for women there is usually a 50:50 chance of either their paternal or maternal X chromosome being switched on. Since the X chromosome contains many genes that are important for immune function, this means that women have a broader range of disease-fighting proteins they can produce.

Hormones

Men and women also have different hormone profiles: from puberty onwards women produce oestrogen, which leads to the expression of female secondary sexual characteristics including breast development and wider hips, while men produce more testosterone. These hormonal differences have a biological impact far beyond the physical changes.

Testosterone and risky behaviour

Testosterone is a hormone produced by the testicles. The sharp rise in testosterone after puberty causes increased muscle development, a larger larynx, a deeper voice and the appearance of facial hair. It also has some effects on the brain, and is associated with risk-taking behaviour and violence. Men consistently underestimate risks, such as driving while intoxicated or climbing on a steep roof without a harness, which is why they are far more likely to suffer accidental death. Since 1942, men aged 20–50 in the wealthiest countries of the world, which include the USA and many countries in Western Europe, are more than twice as likely to die compared to women. The most common cause of death among this group is unintentional injury.

Men are also much less likely to seek help for mental health conditions, which is also a likely contributor to increased rates of substance abuse and subsequent risky behaviour. One important caveat here is that it is very difficult to pick apart how much of this is due to differing social norms for behaviour and how much is due to hormones. Many of these gender-based behaviours are learned and preventable, rather than the direct result of hormones acting on the brain.

Oestrogen's protective role

Urban Dictionary describes the 'man cold' as a 'true terrible, debilitating disease' that will be fatal without 'large amounts of mindless TV' while the afflicted man is provided with endless cups of tea and chocolate biscuits by a caring woman. Although we tend to laugh at the stereotype of men suffering more from such afflictions, there is an underlying truth to it. Oestrogen is associated with an increased ability to conquer viruses by impairing their ability to reproduce, meaning that the increased symptoms that men complain of probably are based in reality.

Oestrogen may also help protect women against heart disease prior to menopause. Women seem to get cardiovascular disease ten years later than men – the rates of cardiovascular disease for women only rise after menopause, which may be due to the reduced levels of oestrogen at this stage. There have been some conflicting studies regarding hormone replacement therapy (HRT) and cardio-vascular disease. Observational studies (which means researchers just measure factors of interest without any intervention) suggested there might be cardiovascular protection. When this was tested in a randomised controlled trial, the trial was stopped early because of excess risk of breast cancer as well as an increased risk of cardio-vascular disease. However, the average age of participants in this trial was 62, so most of these women were many years past meno-pause, and when the researchers reanalysed the data by age group, there was no extra cardiovascular risk in women in the 50–59 age group. The general consensus is that HRT is safe when it is started around the time of menopause, and it is possible that at this time it may offer some protection against cardiovascular disease, but in women over 60 probably shouldn't commence HRT. As always, individual treatments should be discussed with your doctor.

Does childbearing influence longevity?

When the Duchess of Cambridge, Kate Middleton, stood on the steps of St Mary's Hospital cradling her healthy baby boy, she must have felt incredible relief at being free of the incessant vomiting and nausea that had plagued her for the past nine months. Although many women vomit during pregnancy, Middleton suffered the rarer and much more severe condition known as hyperemesis gravidarum. In the days before intravenous fluids and anti-nausea medications, women used to die from this condition. Many women with hyperemesis gravidarum can actually weigh less after giving birth than they did prior, but their babies are still a healthy weight, having taken first pass at their mother's kilojoules for the previous nine months.

Pregnancy is a feat of endurance that is up there with the Tour de France. During pregnancy, the placenta implants into the wall of the uterus, giving the baby access to the mother's blood supply so it can take oxygen, fats, glucose, protein, iron, zinc and all the other micronutrients required to form a whole small human. Giving birth can be straightforward, but it can also result in birth-related injuries, such as tearing of the muscles of the pelvic floor and nerve damage. If a woman chooses to breastfeed, this uses an additional 2000 kilojoules a day. This physiological load is the likely reason why women who have had more children are more likely to be frail.

Women who have had children also have shorter telomeres, which are the caps on the end of chromosomes. As we saw in chapter 2, shorter telomeres are associated with an earlier risk of mortality. However, it is important to remember that this study only looked at one point in time, like a still frame from a movie, so it does not mean that these women necessarily had reduced life expectancy – we can only know this with further research. This is also balanced by the decreased risk of certain cancers, such as breast, ovarian and uterine, that is seen in women who have had children.

In past centuries, pregnancy and birth were incredibly risky for both mother and child, and each labour had a realistic chance of ending in death for both. This meant it was difficult for early researchers to determine the relationship between the number of children born and a woman's life expectancy. In a historical analysis of English aristocrats, the researchers found a clever way to work around this. They looked only at women who lived beyond the age of 60, and found that the more children a woman had, the lower her life expectancy.

Yet other recent longitudinal studies of parity and survival have some positive findings. Women who gave birth after age 33 had twice the odds of living to 95 years or older than those who had their last child by age 29. Women who gave birth after 40 were also four times more likely to live to 100. Thomas Perls, a professor of medicine at Boston University, said, 'The age at last childbirth can be a rate of ageing indicator. The natural ability to have a child at an older age likely indicates that a woman's reproductive system is ageing slowly, and therefore so is the rest of her body.'

THE EVOLUTIONARY ADVANTAGE OF FEMALE LONGEVITY

Humans and orcas are the only two species where females survive for a significant time after menopause. Although woman in her fifties may no longer be able to bear children, she is very capable of leading an active life. In societies that still follow a hunter-gatherer way of living, these women still contribute actively to the survival of their grandchildren, by helping their daughters gather food to feed their own growing families. It is likely that this prolonged survival past menopause is the result of an evolutionary advantage to future generations. Pregnancy, childbirth and breastfeeding use a huge amount of maternal resources, and human children are also dependent on others for survival for a prolonged period to allow brain development. Compared to other species, human childhood is incredibly long, and in traditional societies adolescents are still learning survival skills, so producing another child at age 60, when you may not live long enough to raise them to independence, is unlikely to lead to an increased number of descendants, but a woman with decades of accumulated knowledge is an incredible asset to a group.

Factors contributing to women's poorer health in old age

There are many conditions that affect women more than men, and that are disabling without being fatal. In the Russian study referred to on page 67, women were more likely to be obese and to have a higher waist–hip ratio, which did not seem to confer the same mortality risk as male smoking, but was associated with poorer physical functioning, possibly due to increased inflammation. Obesity is also a risk factor for sarcopenia and frailty in later years.

Access to health care

Unconscious biases are social stereotypes about certain groups of people that individuals adopt without being aware of them. Many men and women hold these biases about women, and this can actually create a barrier to women seeking health care. Although cardiovascular disease is the leading cause of death for women, women are less likely to be diagnosed with a heart attack than men, and less likely to receive timely care when they do, because heart disease is seen as a problem for middle-aged men. This lack of awareness can actually be deadly, because the longer it takes to receive treatment, the greater the damage to the heart muscle. (See chapter 17 for more about heart disease.)

The historical diagnosis of hysteria, which was largely applied to women, was developed at a time when our understanding of disease and our ability to identify it were rudimentary. Although we now have far more sophisticated diagnostic techniques, the stereotype that a woman's symptoms are 'all in her head' remains.

Gender roles

I have seen ads in women's bathrooms urging them to get their partners to have a prostate check. No man I've asked has seen an advertisement in the men's toilets encouraging them to ask their partners about the new five-year cervical screening test.

Women are expected to care for everyone's health and well-being at the expense of our own. Although this has begun to shift in recent years, women still spend far more hours performing household tasks than men. Even after retirement, gender roles are still shaped in a traditional way in some countries, so while men are free to work on their golf game, women continue to perform the role of a housewife. This unequal distribution of household activities limits women's participation in more active leisure pursuits and other social activities, which may have a negative effect on their health.

Financial inequality

Financial stress also has a significant role in poorer health outcomes for women. The gender pay gap is alive and well, with women consistently earning less than men, even in the same profession, which gives women less money to save. Women are also far more likely to take breaks from their careers to care for children or older parents, which has a significant impact on savings for retirement. In Australia, women who retired in 2016 had an average super balance of $157,000 while men had $271,000. In the USA only

55 per cent of women are now confident about retiring comfortably, compared to 68 per cent of men. This is not surprising when you consider that in 2018 the median income for women working full-time was 81 per cent of the median income for men working full-time. The links between socio-economic status and health are well established – if women are worried about their finances, it is harder to make choices to optimise wellbeing, not to mention the anxiety and stress that accompanies financial insecurity.

Reconsidering self-care

Whether we are mothers or not, women are encouraged to put others first. If we do decide to have children, everything becomes about the baby. During pregnancy we are flooded with advice about taking care of the baby, but not about ourselves. We make our children nutritious meals while eating their leftovers; we take them to sport at the expense of our own exercise; we miss catching up with friends so they can go to yet another birthday party. This is combined with the expectation that we will organise the household and look after everyone else's health. It is little wonder that by the time the children are grown, this has become so ingrained that we forget to question our priorities.

Following rigid gender roles is bad for everyone: it means men are more likely to die young, while women suffer poor health. Thankfully, these stereotypes seem to be shifting. Many men now expect to play a far more active part in caring for their children than their fathers ever did. It is also becoming more acceptable for men to express their fear and sadness, rather than masking these feelings with anger or alcohol.

The challenge for each of us is to consider what self-care means and how we can prioritise it on a day-to-day basis. It is lovely to have a spa day occasionally, but this will not create health without adequate nutrition, sleep and exercise. The first step in self-care is believing that you are worthy of kindness and compassion, and using this principle to guide everyday decisions. This can include examining the division of household chores so that both spouses have time for leisure, saying no to a late night babysitting grandchildren if you need to catch up on sleep, or deciding that your daily walk with a friend is a non-negotiable part of your routine.

PART 2
CREATING HEALTH

7

WHAT IS HEALTH?

*The purpose of 'being healthy' is not health itself, it is
what health allows us to do.*

Have you ever thought about what it really means to be healthy?
The most reductive definition is the absence of disease, but
this is a narrow and restrictive definition. The World Health
Organisation defines health as complete physical, mental and
social wellbeing, would exclude anyone with a chronic disease,
including the multiple Olympic athletes competing who have
chronic diseases such as asthma or diabetes. In fact, by the age
of 65, around 60 per cent of us will have a chronic disease; this
does not preclude an active, vibrant and long life. A study of
centenarians found that almost half had been diagnosed with an
age-related chronic disease prior to age 80. A new diagnosis does
not have to be the beginning of the end. Also, health is not a
constant; we all suffer various maladies such as colds and flu that
make us temporarily unwell. Simply being free of disease is not
the same as feeling truly well.

We need to define health as a state of being in which we feel
energised, mentally alert and engaged with life, and can undertake

activities that add meaning and purpose. Health is something we create and enjoy in the present. It is something we can achieve now. As I mentioned in the introduction, research has shown how simple day-to-day choices about what we eat, how we move and what social and leisure activities we undertake not only fill us with vitality but also contribute to longevity. In the following chapters I will explore the daily lifestyle choices that can reduce the risk of chronic disease and slow the rate of age-related change, as well as the ways that they have benefits right now. You may well have heard of some of them, but I'm hoping that explaining some of the research behind them will inspire you to implement change.

THE CASE AGAINST SMOKING

It seems likely that most people reading a book like this will be non-smokers, but just in case you or a loved one still smoke, here are some sobering statistics:

Smoking increases the risk of lung cancer by around 30 times, as well as the risk of dementia, heart disease, breast cancer and stroke.

Smoking is also linked to cervical cancer, oesophageal cancer, head and neck cancer and bowel cancer.

Cigarette smoke is a mixture of approximately 5000 chemical compounds, of which several dozen are carcinogens, co-carcinogens, mutagens and tumour promoters. This means that smoking will increase the risk of DNA damage. Smoking is also linked with accelerated ageing overall.

Even if you do not develop cancer, smoking puts you (and your non-smoking loved ones) at risk of developing chronic obstructive pulmonary disease (COPD) due to scarring and narrowing of the airways in the lung. Rather than making it hard to breathe in, COPD causes difficulty in breathing out, which can lead to some air becoming trapped. This can damage the alveoli, which are the small sacs in our lungs where the oxygen and carbon dioxide exchange takes place. Over time they can break down, which means that there is less of the lung to access oxygen in the air and to release carbon dioxide.

One of the most important things to know about smoking is that it is never too late to quit. Even people who quit in their seventies can still enjoy survival benefits, although the sooner you give up the cigarettes, the sooner the damage stops.

If you are a smoker, stopping is likely to be the most meaningful thing you can do for your health. I would suggest making an appointment with your doctor to help you with this today.

8

NOURISHMENT

*Food is something that enhances our lives. Whether we're
eating alone or sharing a meal with others, it is an act
of self-care.*

Our nutritional needs change throughout our lives, and this
continues to be true in older age. While the optimal nutrient
profile for someone aged 30 may not have the same health benefits
for someone aged 80, many studies show that a Mediterranean
approach to food has long-term benefits to both physical and
cognitive health at all stages of life. Along with a high intake of
plant-based foods, fish and olive oil (and a low intake of processed
foods and red meat), a key aspect of this approach is to recognise that food is something to enhance your life and share with
others, not something we deny ourselves in the hope of a long-
term benefit.

I frequently see older people who are struggling because they
are malnourished. The thing is, I don't work in a particularly
deprived area. These people are not rich, but they have a house
and enough income to buy food. But, often through lack of knowledge or as a result of isolation, they are choosing foods that are not

optimal for their health. Sometimes it is simply that they can't be bothered making anything more than tea and toast for themselves.

Educating people about nutrition is one of my most important health interventions. I spend a lot of time thinking about food. I avidly seek out the latest research on nutrition – both the large population studies and the smaller interventional trials. I think a lot about what constitutes a well-rounded diet.

As a foodie, I also think a lot about how much I enjoy the meals I create. I love to combine flavours and textures, to make things that are new and interesting. When I have some extra time, I find it incredibly relaxing to hang out in the kitchen and cook. I am my own favourite person to cook for.

I have read many health books (and Instagram posts) promising amazing benefits from consuming just one so-called 'superfood' – claims like 'broccoli kills cancer cells'. What the authors fail to mention is that the research was conducted in a test tube using phytochemicals extracted from the broccoli, and that to get the equivalent dose, we'd need to eat 10 kilograms of broccoli! The truth is, there is no such thing as a superfood: kale has a lot of health properties, but if that's all you ate, you would end up with some life-threatening dietary deficiencies. Then there are the countless jars of vitamins, minerals and other supplements made from various plant extracts. Study after study has shown that the only thing most dietary supplements do is create expensive urine.

Nutrition basics

Nutrition is one of the most confusing and fraught areas of healthy living. The sheer number of diet books available is overwhelming. There are also many people with no health qualifications giving nutritional advice that is at best wrong and is in some cases actively harmful. The reality is that nutrition science is, like any branch of science, extremely complex, but there are some simple basic truths. Understanding the basics of nutrition is the first step to making informed decisions for your own health.

Macronutrients

To put it simply, macronutrients are the components of our diet that make up the bulk of our food and provide energy. They are divided into three groups: carbohydrates, fats and protein. Our carbohydrate and fat needs don't change significantly through the lifespan, but our protein needs do, depending on growth and rates of muscle breakdown.

Carbohydrates

In chemical terms, carbohydrates are small or large molecules made of carbon, oxygen and hydrogen that can be broken down by our bodies to provide energy. The smallest carbohydrate molecule is a monosaccharide. Carbohydrates can be simple (composed of only one or two monosaccharides), often referred to as sugars, or complex (made of chains of monosaccharides), which include fibre and starch. Starch is actually the way plants store carbohydrates for energy, while fibre is part of the structure of plants. The small molecules glucose, fructose and sucrose taste sweet to us and are absorbed rapidly in the small intestine. The complex carbohydrates take longer to digest, and we can't digest fibre with our own digestive enzymes at all, instead relying on our friendly gut bacteria to do the job for us.

Our brains rely on a ready supply of glucose for energy, as this is the preferred energy source. We constantly have glucose circulating in our blood, and this is kept in a tightly regulated range;

if it is too low our cells can't function properly and if it is too high it can damage many tissues. (Elevated blood glucose levels occur in diabetes and can have many harms – see chapter 19 for more about this.)

Even if we haven't eaten for a while, we need to have a ready supply of glucose. To achieve this, we have stores of glycogen in the liver and muscles which can easily be converted to glucose as needed. However, we are only able to store enough glycogen for one to two days' worth of energy, so we also store energy as fat. Glycogen can be converted to glucose very quickly, but it takes a little longer for fat to become available to be used for energy. When someone is doing short, sharp bursts of activity, such as sprinting or lifting weights, glycogen provides a readily accessible supply of glucose. For a longer period of activity, like going for a run, there is time for our bodies to start breaking down fat stores and using fatty acids as an energy source.

Fats

Lipids, or fats, are another essential building block of life. As well as being a source of energy, they also have essential roles in the structure and function of cells. Lipids form part of our cell membranes and are also needed to make hormones such as oestrogen. They form a protective coating around nerve cells, help to insulate our bodies and are part of the oil our skin secretes to protect us from water.

Humans can synthesise fat from sugars in the diet, but we cannot synthesise all the types of fats that we need (the essential fatty acids: linoleic acid, an omega-6 fatty acid; and alpha-linoleic acid, an omega-3 fatty acid). This means that the type of fats we eat can affect the structure of our cells and some of the hormones that help our cells communicate, which in turn affects how well they function.

One controversial topic in nutrition is saturated fats. These are fats that come predominantly from animal sources and have been demonised as the main cause of heart disease. The fat itself doesn't block the arteries, but it can lead to higher levels of blood cholesterol and low-density lipoprotein in the blood, both of which contribute to the development of vascular disease. There is ongoing controversy about whether saturated fat really is a primary driver of heart disease. Similar to other macronutrients, the whole diet is probably far more important than one macronutrient.

Further problems ensued when we were told to replace butter with margarine, avoid fatty meats, choose low-fat milk, cream and yoghurt and use only vegetable oils. Most 'low-fat' foods were higher in sugar to compensate for the reduced flavour and feeling of satiety. Proving causation is challenging, but rates of obesity and chronic disease continued to rise along with the tidal wave of low-fat foods.

Another result of the advice to avoid animal fat to cut down on saturated fat was the rise of trans-fats. Many vegetable oils are liquid at room temperature, through a chemical process that involves adding more hydrogen atoms, these become solid at room temperature. Oils that are completely hydrogenated essentially become saturated, which defeats the purpose of replacing animal fats with vegetable sources, so manufacturers used partial hydrogenation instead, which creates trans-fats. These fats were widely used in the processed food industry as they increased the shelf life of pies, biscuits and so on. However, we now know that trans-fats not only increase LDL cholesterol (the bad kind), but reduce the good HDL cholesterol, and they have been banned in the USA, Canada and parts of Europe. In Australia, manufacturers must include trans-fats on the nutrition information panel, but they are not yet banned.

Protein

A protein is a chain of amino acids, which have a wide variety of uses in our bodies. They form part of the structures of our cells, they can act as enzymes to speed up biochemical reactions and they can help to regulate cellular functions. As well as being made of a specific sequence of amino acids, proteins fold to form a specific shape. The bonds between these folds are weaker than those in the chain, and so are more sensitive to outside influences.

Our protein needs change over the lifespan; we have different requirements at different stages of life. Not surprisingly, growing children need more protein per gram of body weight, but what might be surprising is that a higher protein intake in early to mid-adulthood might actually speed up mortality. Observational studies have shown that in adults aged under 65, mortality is higher with a higher protein intake, which is unfortunate news for would-be beefcakes trying to get the biggest biceps they can. This relationship reverses after the age of 65, when a higher protein intake is associated with lower mortality, largely because it protects against muscle breakdown, allowing people to stay active for longer, with all of the benefits that exercise brings (see chapter 9).

If you include some dairy, eggs, meat, fish, nuts, seeds or legumes with each meal, you are almost certainly getting enough protein.

WHAT IS KETOSIS?

The ketogenic diet is a recent dietary trend, with advocates claiming all sorts of health benefits, including weight loss, decreased risk of type 2 diabetes and protection against dementia. The ketogenic diet involves an extremely strict reduction of carbohydrates, which are replaced with fats. Over the course of a few days, the body uses up the glycogen stores and this leads to a metabolic shift, driven by the depletion of carbohydrate availability. This will decrease levels of insulin and increase another hormone called glucagon, which normally stimulates the release of glucose from the glycogen stores. This low insulin/high glucagon ratio, along with the hormone lipase, leads to the release of fat stores into the blood as fatty acids, which then travel to the liver to be converted to ketone bodies.

These ketone bodies become an alternate fuel source for mitochondria, including in the brain. Ketone bodies will start to be produced after fasting for 12–14 hours. People on a ketogenic diet aim to limit carbohydrates to less than 50 grams per day so their bodies keep producing ketone bodies. This means basically excluding almost all carbohydrate-containing foods, including vegetables that grow below the ground and wholegrains.

There are some medical uses for this diet, such as in patients with refractory epilepsy, and some obesity physicians are using this for weight loss, because ketosis does suppress appetite. However, although there are many health claims associated with this diet (often from animal studies), the restriction on eating vegetables and wholegrains means that a ketogenic diet is often very low in fibre, which is linked with many adverse health outcomes. While some short-term studies show some metabolic benefits, such as positive changes in blood lipid profiles, there are no long-term studies showing actual preventative outcomes. In addition, this is an incredibly restrictive diet. This means that every meal needs to be carefully planned, and going out for a casual pizza with friends is off limits. Personally, I don't think this is a price worth paying.

Micronutrients

Micronutrients are the minerals and vitamins we need in small amounts for our bodies to function. Minerals include iron to make the oxygen-carrying molecules in red blood cells; zinc to make many of the enzymes that are catalysts for the chemical reactions; and calcium to make bone cells and assist in cellular signalling. Vitamins include vitamin K, which plays a role in blood clotting and bone health; vitamin C, which is part of collagen and essential for tissue integrity; and vitamin D, which is important for calcium metabolism and therefore bone health.

Although it can seem like more is better, when it comes to vitamins, it is actually important to get just the right amount: not too little, not too much. Some vitamins can be toxic if too much is consumed. Basically, once you have enough, there is no benefit to extra.

A NOTE ABOUT NUTRITION RESEARCH

To fully appreciate nutrition advice, it is important to have some understanding of where this evidence actually comes from.

Many studies of nutrition are observational, meaning researchers periodically collect data about eating habits and health outcomes from a group of people without testing a particular dietary intervention. These studies have given us invaluable information about nutrition habits and longevity, but one of the challenges with this type of research is that pro-health behaviours don't occur in isolation: someone who is health conscious in one aspect of their life is likely to be health conscious in another. This means that people who are able to eat better are more likely to exercise and to undertake other health strategies, so it can be hard to tease out what is the most important factor.

A more rigorous study design is a randomised controlled trial (RCT), where participants are randomly divided into two groups and given differing interventions. The participants are recruited as one group, then randomly assigned to either an intervention arm or control arm (this might be a placebo or a different treatment). If randomisation has been conducted properly, the groups should be well-matched, and any differences should be the result of the intervention. RCTs are usually based on information from an observational trial, which the researchers use to develop a hypothesis. RCTs are hard to do in nutritional research, because unless people are kept in controlled conditions, they are unlikely to completely stick to any diet. There have been some trials that have gone for a few weeks and have done exactly this, but they are only short-term and only involve small numbers of people, because they are very expensive. There are some large RCTs that go for longer in the community, but without the same level of control over the participants.

While we still have a lot to learn, we have enough consistent data to know the optimal dietary patterns for good health.

A short history of dietary advice

From the 1960s onwards, people were told that the way to control weight was to eat as little fat as possible. At the time, this seemed to make sense because fat has more kilojoules per gram than protein or carbohydrates (37 kilojoules per gram versus 17 kilojoules).

Even today, low-fat dairy is still recommended in many nutrition guidelines despite there being no evidence that choosing low-fat over regular improves health outcomes. Low-fat dairy products, in particular yoghurt, often have large quantities of added sugar to make them more palatable, and easier to overeat. At a societal level, throughout the decades when low-fat diets were promoted, obesity continued to rise.

The current demon macronutrient is carbohydrates, but carbohydrates are a broad group, and are digested and absorbed at hugely different rates. Most of the kilojoules in both brown rice and soft drink come from carbohydrates, yet the rice is digested slowly (releasing glucose, vitamins, amino acids and minerals into the bloodstream and also feeding the microbiome), while soft drink provides a massive sugar rush and nothing else.

Other diets exclude entire food groups (such as dairy or grains). Many people are drawn towards veganism for health benefits, but without self-education and careful consultation with a dietician, there is a real risk of developing nutrient deficiencies, such as B12 and iron.

One of the most important things we can do for our nutrition is to eat a large variety of foods. In most cases, excluding a specific macronutrient or food group is unnecessary, and won't improve health.

The Mediterranean diet

People who live around the Mediterranean Sea have been trading for millennia, so have developed many shared dietary patterns, including the use of olive oil in cooking, a preference for fish and seafood rather than red meat, and the consumption of a wide variety of plant foods. Some of the islands in this region, where people still follow these traditional diets, are now home to some of the longest-lived populations in the world, and this way of eating seems to play a large role in this longevity (along with strong social connections, daily physical activity and other lifestyle factors).

In 2013 the PREDIMED Study was published in the *New England Journal of Medicine*. The researchers recruited more than 7000 people in Spain and randomly assigned them to either a Mediterranean diet (with two streams, one supplemented with olive oil and one with nuts) or a control diet. People on the Mediterranean diet were encouraged to eat the following foods:

- vegetables and fruits
- olive oil
- nuts
- legumes
- fish
- sofrito (a tomato sauce made with garlic and onion)

They were discouraged from consuming soda, commercially baked goods and red and processed meats.

The control diet was based on lean meat, seafood, pasta, potatoes, bread and low-fat dairy.

The trial was stopped early (after 4.8 years) because the survival differences were already statistically significant for mortality, with 3.8 per cent of people on the Mediterranean diet with olive oil dying, 3.4 per cent of those having the Mediterranean diet with nuts dying and 4.4 per cent in the control group dying. This may sound small, but it meant those in the Mediterranean diet group had a one-third reduction in mortality, even after just a few years. This effect was even stronger in those who had better adherence.

There are similar findings among migrants from these areas who have continued their traditional dietary patterns. One of the best studied is the Greek diaspora in Melbourne. Professor Catherine Itsiopoulos has studied this group extensively and found that despite living in the suburbs of a large city, rather than on an idyllic island, their eating patterns still offered protection from cardiovascular disease relative to other Australian populations.

Why plant-based foods are so good for you

Countless studies have found positive health outcomes associated with high intakes of unprocessed or minimally processed plant foods. These include vegetables, fruits, legumes, nuts, and wholegrains such as freekeh or barley.

They're high in fibre

The first reason plant foods are so good for us is that they tend to be high in fibre (the cellulose and other starches that we can't digest because we lack the right enzymes). Fibre not only slows down absorption from the small intestine (preventing blood sugar spikes), it also helps us feel fuller for longer. And our gut bacteria love fibre. They are able to break it down into its components, providing us with additional nutrients and helping to attract water to the colon, which helps prevent constipation.

The average Australian adult eats around 20 grams of fibre per day, less than the recommended 25–30. In a study published in *The Lancet* in 2019, people with the highest fibre intake had a 15–30 per cent decreased risk of death. A high-fibre diet was shown to decrease the risk of cardiovascular disease, bowel cancer, breast cancer and diabetes.

They are loaded with micronutrients

It is not just the fibre in plant foods that has a huge impact on health. Plant foods contain multiple different nutrients. For example, an orange is a vehicle for a seed. These fruits often evolved so animals would eat them and then hopefully poo them out in a good growing spot, far from the parent tree. When we eat an orange, we get multiple types of fibre, a variety of bacteria, and vitamins that we need for body function but can't make ourselves, like vitamin C. Plants are good sources of vitamin A, K and E, too. They also contain compounds called polyphenols, which give them the colours, scents and flavours that attract particular insects and birds for pollination or seed dispersal, or protect them against UV radiation or predators. Some polyphenols also have a role in cell growth and repair for plants. Just as these compounds are part of the plant's chemical defence against DNA damage, they have the same effect in our own cells. Foods rich in polyphenols include blueberries, dark chocolate, tea, spices, nuts, coffee and olive oil. High intake of phenolic-rich fruits, vegetables and wholegrains reduces the risk of cancer, cardiovascular disease, chronic inflammation and metabolic disorders.

Less room on the plate for meat

Eating more vegetables also generally means there is less room in the diet for meat. Processed meats such as ham, bacon, salami and hot dogs are unequivocally associated with an increased (albeit small) risk of bowel cancer. The cause isn't completely clear, but it might be due to the heme protein, which gives red meat its red colour, or to nitrate-based preservatives, which can form harmful compounds, particularly when they are heated. Diets high in red meat may also increase the risk of bowel cancer, although this is less definitive.

One of the difficulties in interpreting the evidence about meat consumption is that the studies often compare people at the extremes of the meat-eating spectrum. There is a big difference between making meat the focus of breakfast, lunch and dinner and consuming a small amount of meat a few times a week. If eating less meat means eating a higher variety of vegetables and wholegrains overall, perhaps it is this higher intake of plant-based food that is providing the benefit, rather the reduced quantity of meat per se. Production methods can also affect the nutritional profiles. For example, pasture-raised beef has a more favourable lipid profile than grain-fed.

After reading many, many studies, I think there is insufficient evidence to justify *completely* excluding beef, lamb, poultry and pork, so I choose instead to restrict my meat intake to one to two evening meals a week. Free-range meat is often more expensive, but as well as having a better nutritional profile, it also often means that the animals have had a better quality of life, which is so important. Meat also uses large amounts of environmental resources, so eating less can help reduce our environmental footprint.

Why ultra-processed foods are so bad for you

According to *Public Health Nutrition*, 'ultra-processed' foods are 'energy-dense, high in unhealthy types of fat, refined starches, free sugars and salt, and poor sources of protein, dietary fibre and micronutrients.' They include many breakfast cereals, savoury snacks, biscuits, confectionary, hot dogs, pies, pizzas, chicken nuggets, instant noodles and many, many more foods.

These highly processed foods are designed to be consumed without ever giving a feeling of satiety, making you crave more and more in order to increase corporate profits. I describe these foods to my children as 'want more foods'. This is why it is possible to eat an entire packet of crackers in one go and still feel hungry.

It is far more meaningful to group foods according to the amount of processing they have had, rather than their biological origin or macronutrient content. As Professor Carlos A. Monteiro and his team have highlighted, grouping foods as grains means putting whole oats (with no added sugar) together with frosted flakes (which contain a whopping 43 per cent sugar). Clearly these foods would have very different effects on your body.

Ultra-processed foods, obesity and chronic disease

Ultra-processed foods are designed to work around your satiety signals, so you just want more and more. This means they are easy to overeat, and so can cause you to consume more kilojoules than you need.

In one trial, a group of people spent two weeks living in and eating only the food they were provided. Half were fed ultra-processed foods and the other whole foods, but with an equal energy and nutrient profile. The group with the ultra-processed foods consistently ate more kilojoules and actually gained an average of almost 1 kilogram in two weeks.

The causes of obesity are complex, and go far beyond individual choice and levels of restraint. Eating patterns are learned behaviours, and they are learned in the context of the environment we live in. If you are hungry and wander into a convenience store, almost all the options available will be ultra-processed foods. Similarly, even though most supermarkets do have a section for fruit and vegetables, the majority of the space is taken up by foods that look nothing like their natural components.

In a study conducted in Spain, researchers recruited more than

22,000 participants and asked them about their diet and intake of ultra-processed foods. They then divided the participants into four groups, based on their intake. Compared to the group with the lowest intake, the group with the highest intake were heavier and were 1.6 times more likely to die during the ten years of study follow-up. (The actual numbers of deaths were small because the average age of the participants at recruitment was 37.6.) This study was published in the same issue of the *British Medical Journal* as another study of over 100,000 people in France, which showed that compared to the lowest consumers of ultra-processed foods, high consumers were more likely to develop cardiovascular disease, in a pattern that was dose dependent. The absolute numbers are small, but the trial only ran for five years and cardiovascular disease takes decades to develop, so it is likely that this gap would widen with time.

These studies are observational, so there is always the caveat that these results could be coincidence, but they are worrying enough to take seriously. Like all foods, these ultra-processed foods are made of a variety of different components and are produced using many different techniques. Whether the problem is the lack of nutrients, high sugar, low-quality fat, lack of fibre or the simple fact that they are so easy to overeat remains to be researched. At this time, I think there is enough evidence to justify making these discretionary foods a limited part of your diet.

Ultra-processed foods and inflammation

Eating highly processed foods is also associated with endotoxaemia (exposure to bacterial products) and a state of low-grade chronic inflammation, which can lead to feeling unwell and lethargic – a bit like having a lingering cold that won't go away. This may be due to increased intestinal permeability and increased exposure to lipopolysaccharides, part of the bacterial cell wall, which induce inflammation. Most of this evidence does come from animals.

Ultra-processed foods are also bad for the microbiome. Not only does the associated lack of fibre mean that the gut microbes don't have as much to eat but the use of emulsifiers, which are very common in ultra-processed food, might have a negative impact on intestinal permeability. In mice, this has been linked with inflammation of the gut, and researchers have hypothesised that this could have a causative role in inflammatory bowel disease, although more research is needed to confirm this.

Ultra-processed foods and the brain

The hippocampus is a region of the brain in the temporal lobe, shaped a bit like a seahorse. In the 1950s, after the hippocampus was removed from patients with epilepsy in an attempt to treat refractory seizures and some disturbing work on animals, it was discovered to have a role in the formation of new memories. The hippocampus is one of the first areas to be damaged in patients with Alzheimer's disease. It is also an area that is particularly sensitive to diet-induced neuro-inflammation, both from high fat and high sugar. It seems that diets high in fats can sensitise the immune cells in this region, which then react more strongly to other immune stimuli, causing inflammation in the hippocampus. This may partly explain the link between diet and dementia.

The hippocampus seems to be so sensitive to the effects of saturated fat and sucrose that a diet high in these can have an immediate negative impact on learning. In one study, 110 healthy lean adults who usually had a healthy diet were recruited and randomly assigned to eat either their normal diet or a diet high in sugars and saturated fats. Because the long-term adverse effects of this diet are well known, the experiment only ran for a few days. The researchers served both groups a toasted cheese sandwich and a chocolate milkshake for breakfast, but these had markedly different nutrient profiles. The 'Western diet' group were also given money and a list of approved fast food options for the rest of the day. The participants also recorded everything else they ate. On the eighth day, the participants on the Western diet performed worse on memory testing, as well as a weakening of appetite control. This study is small and involved younger adults, but it still highlights why it is so important to pay attention to the quality of nutrition on a day-to-day basis. Being able to focus and learn is critical for enjoying life at any stage, and eating well gives you an immediate pay-off.

Food and mood

The right food doesn't just have positive effects on cognition; there is also increasing evidence that it could actually be a treatment for depression. While the PREDIMED study referred to on page 93 wasn't designed to examine mental health, the researchers still found that those in the Mediterranean diet group had better mental health than those in the control diet.

I first learnt about this fascinating area when I listened to a podcast by Professor Felice Jacka of the Food and Mood Centre at Deakin University, who is a founding member of the International Society for Nutritional Psychiatry Research. Professor Jacka has been one of the key instigators into research in this area, and led the first randomised controlled trial looking at the interaction between diet and mental health. The aptly named SMILES trial, published in 2017, recruited 67 people who were being treated for depression and randomised half to seven dietitian visits and half to seven social visits. The dietary advice was, unsurprisingly, to eat lots of vegetables, wholegrains, olive oil and nuts, and to avoid highly processed foods or foods with added sugar. After twelve weeks, the groups who were given dietary advice had decreased symptoms of depression.

Although this is a small trial, the results are very positive. Psychiatric disorders are a significant cause of poor health from adolescence onwards, with 45 per cent of Australians experiencing a mental health disorder in their lifetime. Not all people respond to current treatments, whether that be medication, psychological counselling or a combination of both. Although the study results will need to be repeated in larger samples before the findings can be applied in treatment guidelines, I still recommend that my patients try this, often in conjunction with other treatments including medication where appropriate. There is so much evidence for the physical health benefits from this eating pattern, there is nothing to lose.

WHAT IS A HEALTHY WEIGHT?

Despite recent efforts in the media to reduce our obsession with being thin, having a low body weight is still a key goal for many people. However, weight is an overly simplistic way to measure wellbeing, particularly with age.

Healthy weight is often defined by body mass index, or BMI. However, there is not a clear linear relationship between increased BMI and mortality. Instead, the graph takes a J-shape, with higher mortality at both lower and higher BMI. This is especially important for adults over 65, where the highest survival rates are actually for people who have been labelled 'overweight', with a BMI of around 28.

One criticism of BMI is that it does not measure body composition, and lean muscle mass is an important predictor of health and function in older age. It may be an advantage to be a little heavier in later decades because it helps to preserve muscle mass, which, in turn, helps boost bone strength. (See chapter 21 for more on this.)

I'm not recommending trying to gain weight if you have been slim your whole life. If you are obese, with a BMI of over 30, it may be beneficial to lose weight, but weight loss without sufficient exercise means muscle loss, and for people who already have low muscle mass, this can lead to significant weakness. For older adults who are in the obese range, seeing a doctor with expertise in weight management can be helpful.

It is incredibly difficult to get away from thinness as a goal in itself, and maintaining weight loss is incredibly difficult. A more sustainable approach might be making dietary changes to feel better, rather than for weight loss. I meet so many people who put off allowing themselves to feel good until they hit a certain weight, but weight is only a small part of health. It is far more important to work towards goals that are personally meaningful, rather than to aim for a number on the scales.

The basics of a nutritious diet

Looking at nutrition textbooks, which go into great detail about different types of fibre, plant phenols and fatty acids, can be quite overwhelming. Even dietary guidelines can be hard to interpret, especially if foods are grouped in ways that don't always make a lot of sense, such as lentils with steak because they both contain protein. Overall, I think there is sufficient evidence to recommend eating a largely plant-based diet, including healthy fats like those found in olive oil, nuts and avocado, and avoiding refined carbo-hydrates, highly processed foods and products with added sugar, while also acknowledging that sometimes it's nice to have a piece of cake.

Above all, preparing and sharing food should be a joyful process. I love creating recipes based on new and interesting flavours and also being able to make them quickly. At the end of this book, I have shared some of my favourite recipes for meals and snacks. I hope you enjoy them as much as I do!

Pleasing your tastebuds

We can have a lot of preconceived notions about what particular foods taste like, even when we have never tried them. We can also develop strong preferences based on only a single food exposure. This is partly why preparing new foods can be challenging, especially when you are cooking for others.

Recently I was speaking to a group about nutrition when a woman in the audience spoke up, saying that she was keen to diversify her diet, but her husband just didn't like things like lentils. I wondered if she had considered hiding them in bolognese or soup! If someone gave me a plate of plain boiled lentils, I'd find them pretty dull too. Before deciding a food is not for you, make sure you eat it cooked well! (See page 280 for my recipe for roast chicken and Puy lentils – it's delicious!)

When choosing what to eat, it's important to remember that food is something that enhances our lives. Whether we're eating alone or sharing a meal with others, it is an act of self-care, which means it is not only about the enjoyment of flavour or the feeling of satiety, but also how you will feel an hour or so after you eat. Will you be tired, grumpy and craving sugar? Or will you feel alert, happy and ready to concentrate?

One of my favourite lunches is wholemeal sourdough bread topped with avocado and sauerkraut (see page 295). Not only is it delicious, but the fibre and good fats keep me going for the rest of the afternoon. I usually only need a few nuts as a snack.

I eat this way because I like to feel energised and focused. I am not a puritan, and I do enjoy the odd sweet every now and then, but on a day-to-day basis, I eat not just for taste but also for energy and wellbeing.

MY TOP FIVE HEALTHY EATING AND DRINKING TIPS

I am a busy woman and I like to keep things simple. I love food, and I do look for foods that I will enjoy, but I also need to make the best choices for my health. These are some of my strategies for eating to feel my best.

1. No soft drink or fruit juice

Soft drink is full of empty kilojoules, has no effect on satiety and its consumption is so strongly linked with obesity that some countries have introduced a tax on drinks with added sugar. Fruit juice has a similar amount of readily available sugar – it's better to eat the whole fruit so you get some fibre to slow down glucose absorption. There have been some studies linking diet soft drinks with poor health outcomes, although these do show correlation, not causation. If you're thirsty, drink cold, fresh water. You can always add a slice or two of citrus or ginger, and/or some mint leaves.

2. No refined carbohydrates

When grains such as wheat are refined to make white flour, the bran and germ (the nutritious bits) are removed, leaving only the starch (this is done to lengthen the shelf life).

However, without fibre, refined carbs are quickly metabolised, spiking our blood sugar and insulin levels. Choose 100 per cent wholegrain versions of foods like pasta and bread, and include more legumes in your meals.

3. No added sugar

Don't add sugar to beverages – it soon stacks up. Avoiding it can be tricky, however, as sugar is added to the majority of ultra-processed foods and even some minimally processed ones, such as some brands of yoghurt. Always check the nutrition label. Milk and dairy products should contain no more than 5 grams of sugar per 100 grams (that's the natural sugar content from lactose). If I am going to enjoy something with added sugar, like cake, I will do it consciously and not rely on it to fix my hunger.

4. No eating after dinner

It's easy to reach for crackers or chocolate while relaxing in the evening after dinner, but eating in front of the TV can quickly lead to consuming more than we need. For some people, going to bed with a full stomach can also lead to reflux. Clean your teeth and tell yourself you're done eating (and drinking) for the day. This will help with metabolic control (see fasting on page 106) as well as sleep.

5. Have alcohol-free days

Moderating alcohol intake is particularly important for women, since we are smaller than men, with different body composition, and alcohol affects us more. The recommendations for alcohol intake for women are no more than two standard drinks per day, with at least two alcohol-free days a week and no more than ten drinks a week. Please note that a standard drink for wine is only 100 millilitres, not a full glass. There is no consistent evidence that alcohol has health benefits, and there is no harm from excluding it altogether. Personally I save alcohol for social occasions only.

Fasting

Regular fasting is a dietary concept that has gained significant traction over recent years. This can mean everything from not eating between meals, to intermittent fasting to multi-day water fasts. Its popularity is based on research findings showing that calorie restriction may be protective against cancer and ageing. For example, alternate day fasting was found to increase lifespan in rats and nematode worms. Other animal studies found that fasting removed senescent cells, which, as we discussed earlier (see page 30), may protect against cancer.

While some people find the 5:2 method, with five days of normal eating and two days of fasting per week achievable and enjoyable, this is not for everyone.

Fortunately, it is not necessary to go without food for days to experience the metabolic benefits of calorie restriction. Dr Satchidananda Panda at the Salk Institute in California says that the time we eat determines whether our cells are able to shift into repair and protect mode. All animals have cellular clocks that respond to light and dark: our bodies release certain hormones when it's time to wake up, time to eat and time to go to sleep.

Dr Panda has shown that mice given access to food for a limited time period are protected from certain chronic diseases compared to other mice who have free access to the same amount of food. The same result has also been shown in humans. During the eating period, the body stores the nutrients and uses the energy to grow. During the fasting period, there is an opportunity for the cells to focus on repair.

There is still no definitive evidence showing the optimum length of a daily fasting period, but Dr Panda recommends getting all your eating done within 8–12 hours.

Changing habits

If you are used to eating a lot of sweet, deep-fried and ultra-processed foods, it can be quite challenging to change your habits. Try to remember that this is not about denial, it is about caring enough about yourself to choose foods that taste great and make you feel good.

Keep it simple

It also helps if you take a fairly simple approach to preparing your meals. On busy days I have been known to serve my family scrambled eggs, avocado and frozen vegetables. It's not exactly something you'd put on Instagram, but it is a highly nutritious meal I can prepare in about five minutes.

Don't be afraid of routines

Many recipe book meal plans suggest having a different break-fast every day, but this won't suit everyone. Personally, I like the routine of my daily porridge with fruit, nuts and chia seeds. Once you develop a good habit, it can be a powerful strategy for staying healthy.

Cook up batches

Healthy eating doesn't need to be time consuming or complicated. I like to eat my evening meal early enough to have ample time to digest, and I also cook for three small children, so anything I make needs to be ready in a hurry. Despite these limitations, it is entirely possible to make something highly nutritious in a short space of time, and by making large quantities I can make my life easier.

Don't shop when you are hungry

One of the challenging aspects of changing our diets is being able to avoid the avalanche of highly processed foods in our super-market aisles, petrol stations, cinemas and cafes. It is a constant act of will not to succumb at the supermarket checkout, or to pick up a chocolate bar when paying for petrol. These foods may give us an immediate energy hit, but a short while later, we'll feel flat and tired and will be craving more. Carry some nuts with you, or an apple, if you know you will be tempted. Better still, do your errands on a full stomach.

A SIMPLE LIST OF FOOD STAPLES

One of my key strategies to help me make good food choices is to keep certain staples in the house. I live 500 metres from a wonderful fruit and vegetable shop and a butcher that only stocks pasture-fed meats. I am incredibly lucky to have access to this wonderful fresh food. To quickly turn these supplies into delicious meals, these are the basics I always have in stock.

Pantry/cupboard:
- olive oil
- balsamic vinegar
- white wine vinegar
- rice wine vinegar
- tinned lentils
- tinned chickpeas
- tinned tomatoes

- dark (90 per cent cocoa) chocolate
- garlic
- onion
- nuts
- sourdough bread

Fridge:
- miso paste
- soy sauce
- eggs
- tofu
- cheese
- yoghurt

Freezer:
- frozen vegetables

9

MOVEMENT

The saying 'use it or lose it' takes on a whole lot more meaning in older age.

Physical activity is an incredibly powerful way to enhance every aspect of our wellbeing: physical, mental and emotional. Regular physical activity keeps our bones and muscles strong, allowing us to be independent in older age. It also protects us against chronic diseases such as cardiac disease, cancer and dementia. Even better, when we move our bodies enough to increase our heart rate, the blood flow to the brain increases and there are changes in the neurotransmitters released, giving us that enjoyable exercise high.

PAULA'S STORY

Paula, 72, first started exercising in her thirties. She freely admits that at that time, her decision was driven purely by vanity: she wanted to look slim. Being fit didn't come into it.

Although she continued to exercise regularly, including lifting light weights, a visit to a friend in a nursing home inspired her to up her game. Everywhere she looked, there

111

were women with walking frames. She did not want that for her older age.

This was when she realised that the true value of exercise wasn't about appearance, it was about function.

Paula found a trainer who helped her to improve her strength and taught her proper weight-training techniques. She sees the dollars spent as an investment in her future.

'I can lift really heavy garden pots. I can do really practical stuff, like carry a toddler, things that are useful for life. It is confidence building, knowing that you are strong.'

Paula rarely sees other women in their fifties and beyond at the gym lifting serious weights. As she says, strength is seen as important for men, but it isn't seen as an asset for women. In fact, for women who value their independence it's essential.

Staying strong

Large epidemiological studies have shown again and again that regular exercise decreases your risk of death. For example, a study published in *The Lancet* in 2012 estimated that physical inactivity was responsible for an incredible 9 per cent of deaths worldwide. The researchers defined physical inactivity as doing less than 150 minutes of any kind of exercise per week, which translates to only 22 minutes per day.

Of course, choosing to exercise is not just about living as long as possible: many people are equally concerned about maintaining their independence, and there is a great deal of evidence that exercise helps with this.

A study published in the *British Medical Journal* in 2014 measured the activity levels of 1680 adults aged 49 and older and monitored their development of disability over two years. An age-adjusted analysis found that the most active group had almost half the risk of disability compared to the least active group. Another analysis of the same data looked at people who already had a disability and found that in this group, the most active were still protected against further physical decline. The researchers defined activity as anything that kept people on the move – walking, gardening, doing housework – and found that the average amount of weekly activity in the highest group was 385 minutes, compared to 192 minutes in the lowest activity group.

Clearly, the saying 'use it or lose it' takes on a whole lot more meaning in older age.

Being dependent on others for simple tasks like going to the shops, or even getting up off the toilet, is a confronting thought. Exercise is one of the best ways to ensure you will stay strong in older age.

How exercise slows ageing and prevents chronic disease

The reason that exercise is so incredibly good for us is that it seems to have a direct effect on cellular ageing, immune function and metabolism. These cellular and physiological changes combine to have an incredible effect on our health.

Exercise and cellular ageing

Exercise influences cellular ageing by creating the right conditions to minimise DNA damage. Exercise has been shown to increase levels of our own antioxidants, which can protect DNA. Given then DNA damage accumulates with ageing, this protection is likely to be a strong factor in exercise keeping you young.

When you exercise, this tells the muscle that there is work to be done. It responds by causing the cells to grow bigger by synthesising more proteins. Exercise also leads to changes in how the cells process energy, making them more efficient. One fascinating study published in *Cell Metabolism* looked at different types of exercise interventions in younger and older adults. The most dramatic response was to high intensity interval training, which involves doing short bursts of exercise at maximal level, such as sprinting as fast as you can. The older adults who undertook this sort of training actually experienced changes in their mitochondria that made them look more like the cells of younger people. This is essentially like exercise turning back the clock.

As we saw in chapter 2, telomeres are the protective DNA caps on the ends of our chromosomes that shorten with each cell division. These can be repaired with enzymes, and exercise can help boost this repair.

In a study of 68 people who were carers for family members with chronic disease and who were sedentary and chronically stressed, half were assigned to an exercise intervention and half were put on a waitlist. The intervention was three 20-minute sessions of moderate intensity exercise, which was gradually increased to four to five 30-minute sessions. After 15 weeks, the participants who undertook the exercise intervention had an increase in the length of their telomeres. As a bonus, they also had a reduction in perceived stress levels.

Exercise and immune function

Exercise also has a striking effect on the immune system, which may be why it has such a dramatic impact on the development of age-related conditions. Exercise has complex effects on inflammation. It can cause small amounts of muscle damage, which in turn triggers the release of the anti-inflammatory cytokine interleukin-6 (IL-6). As an illustration of how complex immune function is, IL-6 usually activates inflammation, but when it is released in the context of exercise, it seems to have the opposite effect.

As many age-related conditions are associated with higher levels of inflammation, this might be an important factor in exercise slowing the rate of inflammaging.

Exercise and metabolism

Regular exercise, as most of us know, has positive effects on metabolism. Exercise can also improve sensitivity to insulin and glucose uptake by muscles, which can lower the risk of diabetes. For anyone who has diabetes or impaired glucose tolerance, increasing your activity levels could help to manage your blood sugar levels. In particular, doing a combination of resistance training to increase muscle strength as well as aerobic training seems to have the greatest benefit. If you are on medication for diabetes, it can be useful to speak to a diabetes educator if you have concerns about hypoglycaemia.

Exercise and cardiovascular health

Many large studies have shown that aerobic exercise, the sort that gets you huffing and puffing, is an excellent way to reduce your risk of death and disease. While more exercise is generally better, the mortality benefits seem to tail off after more than 100 minutes a day of moderate to high intensity exercise. Even the 'weekend warriors' who engage in one to two 75-minute sessions of exercise once or twice a week see a mortality benefit.

Aerobic exercise has many positive physiological benefits. It is associated with more favourable blood lipid profiles (the amount of cholesterol and triglycerides in your bloodstream). It can increase insulin sensitivity and help to decrease the risk of type 2 diabetes.

Aerobic exercise can also lower blood pressure. High blood pressure is a huge cause of mortality and heart disease, but making lifestyle changes can reduce blood pressure significantly. Even if you can't stop your blood pressure medications, reducing your blood pressure a little with exercise can still help.

How exercise protects the brain

When we exercise, we don't just wake up our hearts, lungs and muscles, we wake up our brains. In an 8.5-year study of 6622 adults with an average age of 73, the fitter that people were, the more likely they were to score higher on cognitive tests. Other studies have found exercise to be a key factor in the prevention of dementia. A study published in *Neurology* in 2018 followed 191 women aged 30–60 for 40 years. At the time of recruitment in 1968, the women's fitness was measured by testing maximal oxygen uptake, which is a measure of aerobic fitness, on a stationary bike. Throughout the study, the women underwent multiple rounds of detailed cognitive assessment. By the end of the study period, 32 per cent of the least fit women had dementia, compared to just 5 per cent of the fittest women.

Exercise also improves brain plasticity, which is the ability of neurons to form new connections and pathways. This is what enables us to learn new skills. When we attempt to learn a new skill, at first we will be clumsy, but with repetition the skill becomes easier, as our brain strengthens these connections and pathways. People who are fitter have denser neural networks and higher brain volumes.

The areas of the brain that benefit most from exercise are the frontal, prefrontal and parietal lobes. The frontal lobes support executive function, which is the ability to plan and understand complex ideas. This is the part of the brain that is often affected in dementia. A study of 41 people with an average age of 67 showed that a six-month exercise program could improve function in areas of the brain that often show age-related change.

As discussed in chapter 8, the hippocampus is an area of the brain involved in memory that is often shrunken in dementia sufferers. Fortunately, aerobic exercise, like dietary interventions, can also lead to improvements in hippocampal function. In trials where people are assigned to do aerobic exercise, researchers have seen an increase in the size of the hippocampus. This is important because one of the characteristic brain changes in Alzheimer's disease sufferers is shrunken hippocampi.

The likely reason for all these benefits is that exercise can trigger the production of brain-derived neurotrophin factor (BDNF), a cell messenger that encourages the development of neural pathways. This, along with the improved blood flow, is why we see such dramatic effects on brain size and function as a result of simply moving our bodies.

How exercise improves mood

When it is dark and cold and I get up early to go to the gym, I am not thinking about how it will improve my immune system, the blood flow to my brain or my long-term muscle strength. I am looking forward to the rush of energy I feel afterwards, and the calmness and mental clarity I will enjoy throughout the day.

The evidence for exercise as an effective treatment for depression and anxiety is so strong that it is listed as a first-line treatment for mild to moderate cases. Anxiety can be a normal part of life, but when it becomes pervasive and intrusive, it can be very disabling. Many studies have shown that an exercise program can help with anxiety symptoms, with most studies having a program that ran for around ten weeks.

Many of you have probably heard of the 'runner's high', the endorphin rush that comes from a hard workout. The chemical changes in the brain that cause this are complex, and the phenomenon is incompletely understood. In rats, exercise increases levels of serotonin, acetylcholine, dopamine and adrenaline in the brain. In humans, blood levels of dopamine and adrenaline rise after exercise. When we activate, we also release endorphins, which act on the opioid receptors (the same ones as morphine). These can reduce anxiety, as well as helping us get through that slow burn of a long run.

Part of the reason exercise is good for your mood is also psychological. It can be a real boost to self-efficacy to start a challenging physical workout and make it through the mental barriers and physical fatigue to finish. Exercise is also an excellent distraction from any life stress, and the time out from daily activities can help us to mentally refresh.

Exercise strengthens bones

With age there is a progressive loss in bone density, leading to an increased risk of fractures (see chapter 21). When we activate muscles, this sends signals to the bones that they need to get stronger as well.

There used to be concerns that strength training could be risky for people with osteoporosis, but this has been disproven in multiple trials. The Lifting Intervention for Training Muscle and Osteoporosis Rehabilitation (LIFTMOR) trial was conducted in

Australia and published in 2018. The researchers recruited 101 women and randomly assigned them to either an eight-month supervised weights program or to at-home exercises. The group who were lifting heavy weights saw a significant increase in bone density.

There is even evidence that these results actually translate to reduced fracture risk in the long term. In a study of 137 women at risk for osteoporosis in Germany, half were assigned to an exercise program that combined high-impact aerobic training and strength training, and half to a low-intensity at-home program. Sixteen years later, the researchers went back to look at this group. They found that 67 per cent of the intervention group were still exercising, and that they had half the risk of fracture compared to the control group. To put this in perspective, the fracture risk reduction from medication is around a third.

Using exercise to manage osteoporosis requires effort, especially compared to taking a tablet. It means taking active steps to incorporate challenging exercise into your life. Some people may not be able to do this, or may choose not to do this, preferring medication instead. It is still not clear how exercise interacts with the medication and if they would enhance each other or not.

One final thing to remember is that most people who fracture don't actually meet the diagnostic criteria for osteoporosis, so it is never too soon to begin taking steps to improve bone health.

USE IT OR LOSE IT

A 2019 study of 315,059 people aged 50–70 asked participants about their current levels of activity in their leisure time, as well as when they were younger. The researcher identified different activity trajectories, with some people being 'maintainers' who stayed active throughout their lives; others who were more active when they were younger; and some who only started exercising at older ages. Not surprisingly, the people who were consistently active had lower rates of death, but where this study gets interesting is that people who only became active at later ages, after a more slovenly youth, enjoyed the same mortality benefits at older ages compared to people who were consistently active. This study showed that we can't rely on our youthful exertion for future benefits, but also that it is not too late to start exercising and reaping the health rewards.

Why women exercise less than men

Evidence for the benefits of exercise in later life is particularly relevant for women, because from adolescence onwards, women are less active than men. The reasons for this start early and remain strong.

Data from the Australian Bureau of Statistics shows that less than 40 per cent of Australian women aged over 18 are doing sufficient exercise (meaning 150 minutes of moderate to high intensity exercise per week). This figure drops to one in five in women aged 75 and older, compared to one in three men in the same age group.

Part of this difference relates to women's fear about how our bodies are scrutinised in public. A 2017 VicHealth (the Victorian Health Promotion Foundation) survey found that 40 per cent of women feel embarrassed to exercise in public, compared to 26 per cent of men – a fear that starts in the teenage years.

When we have children, we also tend to put their health needs above our own. It can also be incredibly hard to access postnatal physiotherapy for those who have been left with pelvic floor issues, leaving women reluctant to exert themselves for fear of urinary leakage.

Another barrier is that it can be very intimidating to start exercising once we have become accustomed to being sedentary. Many people don't know where to start, or face difficulty due to chronic medical conditions.

The four elements of exercise

The Australian guideline for exercise is 150 minutes a week of moderate to intense exercise. While 30 minutes a day sounds achievable, I find that most people need a bit more guidance than this. To get the best results, there are four elements that should be included.

1. Pelvic floor and core

I see so many older women struggling with the combination of back pain and urinary incontinence, but I also see many women in their thirties who can't run after their children in the park because they are worried they will leak urine.

Your pelvic floor is a sling of muscles that support your pelvic organs. These muscles work in conjunction with the deep core and back muscles to support you through the day. We also rely on our pelvic floor to support continence.

If you are planning to start doing any exercise beyond walking, or if you want to increase the intensity of your current exercise program, this is where you need to begin. Without proper activation of these muscles it is possible to worsen incontinence and back pain. Learning to safely activate and strengthen these muscles is key to getting stronger without injury.

2. Aerobic exercise

This is the exercise that gets us huffing and puffing. When we move, we increase the energy demands on our muscles. When walking briskly up a hill, you might feel your heart beat faster to supply more blood to your muscles, your breathing will become deeper and more rapid, you may start to sweat to help cool your body, and you may feel a burning sensation in your muscles.

If you do this every day, your body will adapt and this will become easier as your muscles grow stronger and your aerobic capacity increases. Aerobic capacity is often measured by how fast your heart beats when you perform an exercise, and how quickly it returns to its normal resting rate. A more practical way to work out if you are exercising with enough intensity is whether or not you can easily hold a conversation. If you can only just get out some short phrases, you're working hard enough. If you are able to easily talk in sentences, it's time to ramp it up.

Aerobic exercise can take any number of forms, from brisk walking and jogging to fitness classes, swimming and bike riding – the list is endless. One effective option is high intensity interval training, which involves alternating high-intensity sprints (running, cycling or swimming) with low-intensity intervals. This can make workouts far more time-efficient, with benefit seen from as little as ten minutes. The key is that the sprints have to be hard, working at maximal intensity, to see the benefit, but for return on time investment, this is an excellent deal. Since it involves working at maximal level, it can be good to check in with a trainer to make sure your technique is right first.

3. Strength training

Strength training (also called resistance training) aims to increase muscle mass and function. Skeletal muscle generates power: the power to sprint, the power to do dead lifts, but also the power to rise from a chair, or to steady yourself if you trip on uneven ground.

Muscle mass decreases with age, and there are also changes in muscle composition. Type I muscle fibres are the ones that are fatigue resistant, but don't generate as much power. Type II fibres generate short, sharp bursts of power. With age, the ratio of type I to type II fibres increases. Fortunately, older adults will experience the same gains in strength through training as younger adults. One study in older men showed that resistance training can lead to an increase in the number of type II muscle fibres, which are also known as fast twitch, and are responsible for producing bursts of power.

Strength training can be done with weights or you can use your own body weight by doing squats and push-ups. Even rising from a chair without using your hands is a start.

In older adults who are frail this is the most effective type of exercise to optimise physical function. For people who want to stay independent well into older age, strength training is the most important thing you can add to your exercise regime. At the same time, it can often be challenging to head to the weights section of the gym by yourself, especially for women. It is possible to injure yourself with incorrect technique, so it is important to get a trainer, or ideally an exercise physiologist, who will make sure you are doing things properly.

4. Balance training

Falls are a common and disabling problem for older adults and are related to decreased balance and muscle strength. Injuries from falls can sometimes be a gateway into needing residential aged care.

Between 30 and 40 per cent of people aged 65 and older will fall each year, and this figure climbs to 50 per cent for those over 80. If you or a loved one has had a fall, or even a near miss or two, it is really important to get assessed by a geriatrician with expertise in this area. There may be reversible factors that your doctor can identify, including poor balance, vision, poor foot sensation, medications and weakness.

The good news is that many studies have shown that exercise can reduce the risk of falls. The optimal exercise program would involve both strength and balance training. This will increase the fast twitch fibres in muscle to allow a quick response to a challenge, as well as improve balance.

One of the best studied methods of fall prevention is Tai Chi, a traditional Chinese practice that is an offshoot of martial arts. It uses very slow, controlled movements that require balance. In one meta-analysis (a summary of all the other studies), falls were reduced by half after 12 months of Tai Chi practice.

There are other simple exercises that can also challenge your balance, including walking heel to toe, stepping side to side or even just standing on one leg. If you feel nervous doing the one-leg stand, start by holding a wall. If any of these bring up problems for you, it would be valuable to see an exercise physiologist or a physiotherapist.

Overcoming the barriers

Fear is one reason people avoid exercise. I know some people are afraid it will be too difficult and they will fail, or they are worried about appearing in public in gym clothes or bathers. If you know you need to start exercising, but are feeling too shy, I suggest finding an exercise buddy. A study of older women enrolled in a strength training program found that they started because they wanted to exercise, but continued because of the social value.

Being unable to find the time is another barrier people often mention for not exercising. If you genuinely want to exercise, make it a priority – include it in your scheduled activities or make a financial commitment, such as paying upfront for group personal training or a ten-week Pilates course. Alternatively, enrol in a water aerobics program or commit to a regular brisk morning walk with a friend, so that you'll go even if you don't feel like it, to avoid letting your friend down.

I manage to include exercise regularly by making it a strict part of my routine. My husband and I have scheduled gym times and we make each other go, even if we don't feel like it. As boring as it sounds, habit and routine are excellent tools for health. Some people will need a different motivator, such as the goal of getting fit for a holiday or being able to lift the grandkids. Keeping out of a nursing home is a pretty good motivator, too.

All the experts I have interviewed say that exercise is an important health strategy that they regularly include in their lives. Among my fellow geriatricians, in particular, you won't find many who are not into health and fitness.

If I were to offer a pill that could make you smarter, happier, stronger and likely to live longer with no side effects, no doubt you would take it. Being active is more work than taking a pill, but the rewards are incomparable. Exercise is an investment in your future, with immediate benefits. Making a habit of movement from today onwards is an essential gift to yourself.

PROLAPSE

It speaks volumes about our society, and the shame around childbirth not going to plan, that women feel too embarrassed to seek help for a problem that affects 30–50 per cent of those over 65. Prolapse is a common condition that is associated with childbirth, particularly if you have had a forceps delivery, as I did for my first child. A vaginal prolapse occurs when the walls of the vagina are weakened and so surrounding structures 'bulge' into the vaginal space. This can be anterior, where the urethra bulges in; posterior, where the rectum bulges in; or it can affect the uterus. It is hard to know how common prolapse is, because many women are unaware they have it until it begins to affect everyday function.

A study of women with an average age of 44 who had routine gynaecological care, around half had some degree of prolapse. Not surprisingly, the more babies a woman has had, the more likely she is to have a prolapse. Anyone who experiences a bulging sensation at the opening of their vagina when they lift weights or run, or who develops urinary incontinence, should see an expert in women's gynaecological health to learn to safely engage their pelvic floor.

If physical therapy isn't enough, some women can also get symptomatic benefit from a pessary, a ring inside the vagina to provide additional support. Surgery can still have a role, but it needs to be considered very carefully.

WHAT IS AN EXERCISE PHYSIOLOGIST?

When I see people in my clinic who would like to start exercise, particularly strength training, most of the time it just isn't appropriate to send them to the local hardcore gym. The reality is that when we are older, we don't recover as well from injury as younger people, and using incorrect technique can be more problematic than ever. In my practice, I usually refer people to an exercise physiologist. An exercise physiologist is a university-qualified allied health professional who is trained to deliver safe and effective exercise interventions. Their training goes far beyond what is required for a personal trainer, meaning that they have a much higher level of knowledge and skill. Starting an exercise program isn't about making quick fixes and gains, it is a lifestyle change that can have a dramatic impact on health and wellbeing, and it is incredibly important to get the right start.

10

SLEEP

Sleep is absolutely critical for normal brain and
body function.

Sleep is literally essential to survival. In fact, *The Guinness Book of World Records* will publish the record for the longest skydive (which involves someone jumping out of a balloon at the edge of space), but will not include records for the greatest number of hours gone without sleep because it is too dangerous.

When we sleep, even though most of our body is not moving, we still burn almost the same number of kilojoules as when we are awake. This is because our brain is busy with vital housekeeping tasks and consolidating learning.

In his book *Why We Sleep*, Professor Matt Walker explains that sleep is the bedrock of our health. Without it, our bodies cannot maximise the benefits of nutrition and exercise. If you think in evolutionary terms, sleep must be really important, given that we still need it despite the danger (we are vulnerable to predators). Research increasingly shows that sleep is absolutely critical for normal brain and body function.

When the evening rolls around and you feel your eyelids

drooping as you sit on the couch, this is your body telling you something important: it is time for bed. Your body has an internal clock, which along with darkness and the cool night air also helps to tell our bodies that it is time for rest. When it reaches evening, your brain releases a hormone called melatonin that helps to induce sleep. Throughout the day, there is also a build-up of a chemical called adenosine in your brain, which is a metabolic by-product of cellular aerobic respiration. This build-up is cleared during sleep, and helps to create sleep pressure, almost as though our brains need a break from the business of the day.

CARRIE'S STORY

When her first child, Abbey, was a little over 12 months old, Carrie returned to full-time work. She felt incredibly guilty and missed her baby terribly. At this time, Abbey started day care, and with this came all the day-care illnesses. For the first month, Abbey had a cold and would cough so much that she would wake herself up, requiring hours of cuddling and feeding to get back to sleep. Carrie's husband tried to help, but Abbey only wanted her mother, who couldn't bear to leave her upset overnight. On the worst nights, Carrie would end up with only four hours of broken sleep.

On those days, she had trouble focusing on tasks at work and felt unproductive. She was grumpy, too – something that did not align with her usual behaviour and values. She also had a continuous run of colds herself.

Carrie couldn't change the run of day-care illnesses, so she looked at what she could change instead. She started going to bed every night at 9, rather than working or watching TV. It wasn't quite the same as getting unbroken sleep, but it kept her functioning until her daughter started sleeping better!

The stages of sleep

When you first drift off to sleep, the first stage is non-REM sleep (REM stands for rapid eye movement). In this stage of sleep, we are still able to move a little. In the next stage, REM sleep, is the stage of sleep when we dream. In this stage, other than our eye muscles, we are paralysed.

Scientists have ways of seeing what is going on in the brain while we sleep. One way is to attach electrodes to the skull to measure the electrical activity of our brain cells. The activity is recorded in waves. Non-REM sleep is divided into three phases: N1, N2 and N3, which show progressively slower, larger waves.

Although we cycle between REM and non-REM sleep throughout the night, longer periods of non-REM slow-wave sleep occur in the earlier parts of the night, gradually becoming shorter until REM becomes the dominant form of sleep.

During REM sleep, our brain waves look similar to when we are awake, but there is a critical difference: other than the muscles that control essential functions, like breathing, we are largely paralysed. If you think back to any dreams you remember, this is for the best: we do not want to go acting out some of the crazy fantasies that occur in our heads during this time! Some people do have a condition where they move during REM sleep, and with their thrashing and kicking, they can actually injure themselves or a bed partner.

Since non-REM and REM sleep occur in different quantities throughout the night, habitually missing sleep at either end can mean that you miss one type of sleep. Since both have different and important functions, this is not good for your brain.

Sleep, learning and memory

Sleep has a key role in learning and memory. In earlier chapters we met the hippocampus, a brain structure involved in creating and retaining new memories that is very sensitive to dietary changes, stress and even exercise. It turns out that the hippocampus also works better after sleep. During sleep, as well as getting rid of the day's brain metabolites, the hippocampus is able to produce growth factors that improve its plasticity. This means that it can develop new connections between cells, or neural networks, which is how we learn.

Sleep allows memories stored in the hippocampus to move to the cortex, where they are more stable. Studies in mice have also shown that during sleep, the brain will run through the day's activities, strengthening the connections between neurons to consolidate these pathways, and moving that information to long-term storage. This also frees up the hippocampus for new learning, meaning that after a good sleep you are better able to absorb new information.

We still have a lot to learn about REM sleep, but one theory is that it may help learning by bringing disparate information together to make connections. This might be why we sometimes wake up with a solution to a troubling problem. Those crazy dreams may be a form of creative thinking that takes place during sleep.

What happens to the sleep-deprived brain?

When we are sleep deprived, not only do we get worse at making memories, we are also unable to focus on tasks. We take the ability to focus on a task for granted, but attention is a higher-order function. Being able to choose a task and stick with it while ignoring distractions is an important part of being a functional adult. Without attention, it becomes very difficult to undertake any kind of task that requires brainpower.

I'm sure none of you would be surprised to read that sleep deprivation also alters our ability to make sensible decisions by affecting the reward circuitry in our brain. This is a group of interconnected structures deep in the brain that respond to stimuli to help us get more of things we enjoy. Basically, any enjoyable stimulus, such as sex, food or being with someone we love, can activate it. It can also be activated by things that are not so good for us, like cigarettes, gambling and amphetamines, because some of the chemicals in those substances can either impact the reward circuits directly, or induce the release of neurotransmitters in this area. These reward-seeking pathways can be tempered by sensible judgement from our higher-order functions, based in the frontal lobe.

When someone is sleep deprived, the reward pathways become more active and the sensible inhibitory part of the brain isn't as powerful. In the research laboratory people have been sleep deprived, then given a gambling task. Those who haven't slept are more reckless with their money because they are seeking instant gratification. We are also more impulsive when we are sleep deprived, meaning that we don't weigh our decisions as carefully. This might be why sleep deprivation is associated with choosing foods that we might otherwise avoid: the sensible part of our brain that might usually stop us eating that cheeseburger for lunch is just not as strong as the desire for the reward.

For anyone who has felt grumpy after a night of poor sleep, you can blame your amygdala. These are a pair of almond-shaped structures on each side of the hippocampus that modulate our emotional response to anything connected to our survival, particularly danger. The neurons in our amygdala become very twitchy when we are tired, so negative stimuli become even more pronounced. This can also explain why sleep deprivation is linked with anxiety.

The effects of chronic sleep deprivation

The benefits of sleep don't end with the brain. Sleep is also essential to help your body function at its peak. Sleep deprivation is a form of bodily stress which, as we saw in chapter 5, triggers cortisol release and inflammation. Chronic sleep deprivation has been linked with a multitude of diseases, including type 2 diabetes, dementia and heart disease. Chronic sleep deprivation is a stress state, leading to changes in brain function and hormone levels that can have serious consequences.

Weight gain

In the previous section, I mentioned that sleep deprivation can affect our decision-making, making us gravitate towards less healthy food choices as a result of overactive reward circuits. There is another way sleep deprivation may lead to weight gain. In the morning at around the time we wake, we have a surge of cortisol to help get us going for the day. Our cortisol levels then gradually fall throughout the day. Being sleep deprived can alter this usual diurnal pattern of cortisol release, having associated knock-on effects on metabolism.

Research has found that sleep deprivation can also lower glucose tolerance. In one study of healthy, slim young adults with normal glucose tolerance, half were woken during the night and half were left to sleep. The next morning they were all tested again, and those who were sleep deprived had poor glucose tolerance – enough to put them into the category of being prediabetic. Ethical considerations prevent researchers from repeating this in the long term to see if participants would become diabetic, but if you already have diabetes, improving your sleep habits is worth a try.

Sleep doesn't just alter how your body handles glucose, it also alters how hungry you are. In a study that I can't believe anyone signed up for, twelve young volunteers were assigned to have either ten hours or four hours in bed and given a continuous infusion of glucose instead of eating to meet all their caloric needs. The researchers took blood samples and found that those with less sleep had higher levels of hunger hormones and lower levels of satiety hormones.

Given that lack of sleep leads to more impulsive food choices, higher levels of hunger and metabolic changes, it seems more than coincidence that the rise in obesity over the last two decades is associated with a drop in the average hours of sleep we are getting. Research published by the sleep foundation in 2016 identified that around 40 per cent of people have problems getting to sleep or maintaining sleep, and this had increased by around 5–10 per cent over the past six years. People who are sleep-restricted for short periods of time, as little as five nights, do put on weight compared to the well-rested comparators.

Chronic disease

Population studies show that people who are chronically sleep deprived have significantly increased risk of developing diseases such as diabetes and heart disease. There is a condition called obstructive sleep apnoea, where the relaxation of the muscles around the throat during sleep causes obstruction of the airway, meaning that people are woken because they can't breathe at least five times an hour, and sometimes many more. Many of these people are undiagnosed and untreated, and not only do they feel pretty rubbish, they also have a much higher risk of chronic disease. If your sleeping partner notices that you snore, snort or appear to stop breathing, or if you just feel extremely tired all the time, it's worth seeing a doctor. Treatment might make you feel so much better.

Shift workers also suffer the adverse effects of poor sleep. In the Nurses' Health Study, a study of nurses over 22 years, those who regularly rotated through night shift had a slightly higher risk of death compared to those who didn't. Those who have done night shift will know there is no way to switch between days and nights without missing some serious sleep. Shift workers get, on average, ten hours less sleep per week than those who work at regular times.

This might not seem relevant if you don't do shift work, but a deficit of ten hours a week is a little over an hour a night – the same as going to bed late and getting up early, which is exactly what so many of us do.

Dementia

When a patient is referred to me because someone suspects dementia, one of my standard questions is about sleep. This is for a few reasons: poor sleep, particularly a change in sleep patterns, can be a symptom of dementia. Lewy body dementia is a form of dementia that has a lot in common with Parkinson's disease, and almost every sufferer will have insomnia and extremely vivid dreams (so vivid, in fact, that they may deny they were dreams at all). Insomnia can also lead to symptoms that mimic dementia, with chronic sufferers feeling foggy in the brain and having trouble concentrating.

When you consider the impact of sleep on memory and learning, it isn't surprising that poor sleep is a risk factor for Alzheimer's disease. The areas of the brain that generate sleep are often the first to show a build-up of amyloid plaque, which is an abnormal protein (see page 209), but we still don't know if poor sleep is the chicken or the egg. It is possible that the build-up of amyloid happens first, and so poor sleep is a symptom of Alzheimer's, but it is also possible that it goes the other way, and the long-term poor sleep contributes to a build-up of amyloid.

One reason poor sleep may cause plaque build-up is because during our sleep, our brain has a chance to do a clean-up from the day's activity. Our brains are surrounded by cerebrospinal fluid, which helps cushion the delicate brain in the hard skull, but also has a role in clearing metabolic waste. During slow-wave sleep, where rhythmic electrical signals flow through the brain, the way this fluid flows around the brain also changes. This is because there is less blood flow, which creates just a little more room around the brain so the fluid is able to get into more places. In a study published in *Science* in 2019, using some very clever MRI techniques, researchers showed that during sleep the pattern of fluid flow changed in synchronisation with the slow brain waves. During sleep, this fluid is better able to bathe the brain cells before it is reabsorbed back into circulation.

This is important because studies of mice have shown that during sleep, this process removes metabolic waste products, including removing beta-amyloid, one of the proteins implicated in the development of dementia. This is thought to be one of the ways that poor sleep is linked to dementia.

In another study, this time in humans, 737 participants had

sleep measured over ten days and a cognitive assessment once a year for an average of 3.3 years. Ninety-seven of the original participants developed dementia, with the people who had the most fragmented sleep being 1.5 times more likely to develop it. It is worth remembering that the sleep was measured via an activity tracker on the wrist, so we don't have detailed knowledge of what was going on in the brain, but it is a tantalising hint that taking steps to prioritise sleep may be a step towards preventing or delaying dementia. The short average length of the follow-up also means that some of these people could have been in a preclinical stage of dementia at the time of enrolment.

The weight of evidence definitely supports adequate sleep as a way to prevent dementia, although like most things in medicine, the relationship between sleep and dementia is complex and seems to go both ways.

Poor immune function

People who sleep less have higher levels of circulating inflammatory markers in their blood. One fascinating study measured people's antibody response to the flu vaccine and compared the results to the amount of sleep they'd had the night before. The researchers identified that people with less sleep had lower antibody titres following the vaccine, meaning they didn't respond as well.

Since sleep deprivation is a physical stress, it is not surprising that shorter sleep also results in less opportunity for cellular repair. In 434 adults who were part of an English cohort, men who reported less sleep had shorter telomeres. In another study where most participants were women, poor sleepers had shorter telomeres in certain cells of the immune system, although this relationship may also have been partly due to higher levels of stress.

This link between telomeres, inflammation and sleep is not quite a smoking gun. We need longer-term studies looking at sleep and frailty, but it is very plausible that adequate sleep gives our cells an opportunity to repair themselves. Personally, I'm not going to let the lack of longitudinal data on this one stop me from getting a good night's sleep!

Do we need less sleep with age?

When babies are first born, they sleep for 16–18 hours a day, although not always when their parents would like! Not surprisingly, given the incredibly rapid pace of physical and mental development, babies and children need more sleep than adults. By the time we reach adulthood, our need for sleep settles at around 7.5–8.5 hours a night, and this remains stable throughout life. So although sleep problems become more common with age, we still need just as much sleep.

So why is harder to sleep as we get older? There are two main reasons. The first is that from our mid-twenties onwards, for unknown reasons, we gradually lose the ability to enter the deepest stage of slow-wave, non-REM sleep, so our sleep is 'lighter' and we are more prone to night-time awakenings. This reduction in slow-wave sleep may also explain some of the metabolic changes associated with sleep. During slow-wave sleep, we release growth hormone. Production of this decreases in line with the reduction of slow-wave sleep through the decades. Less slow-wave sleep means that the trough of cortisol is less profound, which may also contribute to nocturnal awakenings.

Another change with older age is that there can be a shift in our circadian rhythm, meaning we feel sleepy earlier than we would like. For those of you who can't watch TV in the evening without nodding off, it's not your fault, it's your body clock. The brains of older adults release their surge of melatonin around an hour earlier than younger adults, often accompanied by a drop in body temperature to get your body ready for bed. This can cause problems with sleep, as it can lead to a nap in an armchair in the early evening, which takes away some of the sleep pressure when you actually want to go to bed. In turn, a frustratingly early waking time follows. This earlier circadian clock is problematic because it doesn't fit with our social habits.

With age, there are also changes in sex hormone levels. Many women report trouble sleeping at the time of menopause, when there are big fluctuations in hormone levels. This can cause night sweats, or 'tropical holidays', as my mother liked to call them. For some women, these are very disruptive at night. There is an increased risk of depression around the time of menopause, too, which can also impact sleep. The good news is that this effect wears off once our bodies become accustomed to the lower hormone levels.

These changes in sleep usually level off at around the age of 60. Many of the sleep issues experienced with age can be improved with lifestyle changes.

Insomnia

There is an important distinction between insomnia and inadequate sleep opportunity. Insomnia is a medical condition where, despite adequate time allocated for sleep, the sufferer takes longer than 30 minutes to fall asleep or wakes earlier than desired and can't get back to sleep. Insomnia can be short-term and triggered by a stressful life event, such as job loss or a relationship breakdown, or it can continue for much longer.

Insomnia is often linked to other medical conditions, particularly depression and anxiety. This makes sense, because anxiety leads to overactivity of the sympathetic nervous system, which is hardly the right state for sleep. Anxiety will often worsen insomnia, but poor sleep can also trigger anxiety. Insomnia can also be triggered by certain medications, such as glucocorticoids or diuretics. Some medical conditions can also interfere with sleep, such as restless leg syndrome, which is almost an ache that needs movement to relieve it.

If you think you might have insomnia, or another medical condition contributing to poor sleep, seeing your doctor is a good start, and perhaps getting a referral to a sleep physician for further investigations.

Treatment for insomnia

Insomnia affects around 10–15 per cent of people, and is more common in women and older adults. The treatment for insomnia with the most evidence to back it up is cognitive behavioural therapy (CBT). CBT aims to help a person identify and challenge unhelpful thoughts and to learn practical self-help strategies. These strategies are designed to bring about positive and immediate changes in the person's quality of life. CBT is usually delivered by a psychologist and involves learning about good sleep habits and strategies to apply them.

CBT for chronic insomnia will involve education about good sleep habits, along with behavioural techniques to develop these. This can actually start with restricting time in bed to build up sleep pressure. The person with insomnia records the number of hours slept, and that is how long they spend in bed, meaning they may only spend five or six hours in bed. This seems counter-intuitive, but it can help to rebuild confidence in the ability to fall asleep. Over time, this is lengthened while also working on other lifestyle aspects to improve sleep duration and quality. The great thing about this as therapy for sleep is that it provides education and life tools that keep working long after the therapy sessions are over.

AVOID SLEEPING TABLETS

If you suffer from insomnia, it can be tempting to reach for a sleeping tablet, but in the long run this is a very bad idea. The most widely used group of sleeping tablets are benzodiazepines (brand names include Valium and Xanax). These act on the brain by increasing the effect of GABA (a neurotransmitter that slows down the activity of the central nervous system and the messages travelling between the brain and the body). Benzodiazepines, which are sedatives, will decrease the time it takes to fall asleep and, depending on the particular brand, can increase the time you remain asleep. However, the brain quickly becomes used to them, meaning that you need higher doses for the medication to work and can suffer withdrawal if you try to reduce them.

When benzodiazepines were first developed in the late 1970s, they were touted as being extremely safe and were very widely prescribed. To this day I still see older adults who have been dependent on them for decades and find it incredibly hard to stop taking them because of withdrawal symptoms. If people are on high doses for a long time and stop suddenly, they can actually have severe withdrawal symptoms and even seizures. Over the long term, the use of benzodiazepines is also associated with an increased risk of dementia. There are similar risks for other sleeping tablets that work on different brain receptors called the Z-drugs. I do occasionally prescribe sleeping tablets for my patients so they can get some rest in the terrible sleeping environment of the hospital, but they are not a solution to long-term insomnia.

Improving sleep

While many people suffer from insomnia, it is far more common that people simply don't give themselves enough time in bed. If you have no trouble falling asleep when your head hits the pillow and it's easy to get back to sleep after waking during the night but you feel tired, vague and irritable during the day, you need to make sleep a priority.

In a world where being busy is valorised and people love to declare how little sleep they need, it can go against the grain to make sleep a priority. It's worth noting that two famous leaders who boasted of only getting four hours sleep a night, Ronald Reagan and Margaret Thatcher, both died of Alzheimer's disease. While not everyone with insufficient sleep will get dementia and a small minority of the population genuinely only needs four hours sleep. Realistically, it's probably not you.

Many people with sleep restriction are accustomed to staying up late and getting up early for work and may need some help to change these habits. Here are some tips that will help.

Get enough daylight

This sounds simple, but daylight is essential to setting your body clock. Exposure to daylight suppresses melatonin release and helps us synchronise with nature. This can be particularly useful for anyone who finds themselves dropping off in the early evening.

By going for a walk outside in the late afternoon, you give yourself a chance to suppress your melatonin for a little longer.

Do some exercise

Being physically active during the day is one way to improve your sleep. The problem is that when you are tired, you don't feel like exercising. Try to think of how it will help you sleep, and the boost it will give you through healthy activation of your sympathetic nervous system. Note, it is best not to do vigorous exercise within three hours of going to bed because this can increase sympathetic nervous system activity and core body temperature.

Avoid stimulants

Many of us use coffee, tea and other caffeinated beverages to perk us up after a poor sleep. Caffeine makes us less sleepy by blocking the receptors for adenosine, which normally drives sleepiness. The problem with caffeine is that it hangs around in the body for quite a long time. It takes around six hours for half of the caffeine we consume to be metabolised, meaning that if you have a coffee at 3 pm, half that caffeine will still be zinging around your body at 9 pm, when you are trying to wind down. Caffeine also disrupts sleep quality, with an impact on REM sleep. If you are serious about improving your sleep, keep your caffeine for the morning.

Keep cool

As we get ready for sleep, our body temperature starts to drop. This cooling is essential for getting off to sleep. It can be a good idea to turn the thermostat down a little at night. The ideal ambient temperature is around 16–18 degrees Celsius. A warm shower or bath has an unexpected effect: it actually cools you by increasing dilation of blood vessels in the skin, which is why this can be an effective sleep tool.

Turn evening lights down low

Just as daylight wakes us, darkness encourages sleep. In the evening, where possible, lights should be turned down to their lowest level. If you have ever seen a rainbow, you will know that light actually comes in multiple wavelengths, which is why we have colour. The light from handheld devices emits blue waves, which is the light that keeps us awake during the day. The problem is that when we are exposed to this light in the evening, through screens and artificial lights, it confuses our circadian clock and decreases the release of melatonin, making it harder to get to sleep. These devices should be avoided for 1–2 hours before bed. Some people even take the step of installing red lighting for the evening.

Avoid evening snacks

Snacking after dinner not only adds excess kilojoules (most of us are reaching for chocolate rather than carrots at this time), it can also impede your sleep. While there is little definitive research on the timing of eating and sleep, going to bed uncomfortably full is not a good feeling. I'm sure those of you who suffer reflux will be nodding emphatically at this point! In terms of an overall balanced diet and optimising the conditions for sleep, I suggest having dinner two to three hours before bed, and not eating again until the next day.

Have a sleep routine

Just like children, we grown-ups do well with a wind-down before bed. If you are planning to go to sleep at ten, start winding down at nine. This may mean having a bath or shower, reading a book, or doing some colouring or meditation. Some people find it helpful to have a notebook by the bed to write down any pressing things for their to-do list that pop into their heads. Getting into the habit of going to sleep at a consistent time of day helps your body clock stay on track.

Similarly, it is a good idea to get up at the same time every day. This means setting an alarm clock for a chosen time each day, whether it is a weekday or weekend. This can feel cruel if you have had a poor sleep the night before, but for some with insomnia, spending extra hours in bed awake or dozing can worsen the problem.

No alcohol close to bedtime

Who hasn't felt a little drowsy after a glass of wine? This is particularly true if you are already tired to begin with. It may feel easier to go to sleep after alcohol – especially since alcohol is a depressant, meaning it slows your brain down – but alcohol actually stops your brain going into deeper sleep cycles and can impede REM sleep, meaning that sleep after alcohol is less refreshing. If you are serious about wanting to feel more refreshed in the morning, it is best to ensure that your last drink is out of your system before you hit the pillow. So, assuming you are following guidelines and only having one to two glasses, I would suggest stopping at least two to three hours before bed.

Keep your bedroom free of distractions

Our bedrooms should provide an environment for relaxation. They should be a place where we habitually wind down, so our brains come to expect this when we walk in for the night. If we use our bedrooms to check emails or watch TV, this sends mixed signals that the bedroom might be a place for activity rather than rest. Of course, the one exception is sex, which can be an excellent sleep aid in itself!

If you lie in bed for long periods of time trying to get to sleep and worrying about it, one technique is to give yourself a set period of time (say, fifteen minutes) to go to sleep. If after that time you are still awake, get up and do something else, such as colouring or reading, until you feel sleepy again. Then get back into bed and give yourself another fifteen minutes, repeating the cycle until you fall asleep. For people with chronic insomnia, this can seem cruel at first, but over time it is a way to create a strong mental association between sleep and your bed.

No napping

I frequently hear from older adults that they just can't fall asleep at night, but consistently doze off in front of the television after dinner. This short sleep is enough to reduce the sleep pressure, so when they want to go to bed, they just aren't tired enough. Even napping earlier in the day is a bad idea if you are sleeping poorly at night. In the evening, it may be better to try another activity that is more engaging than TV, such as going for a gentle after-dinner walk.

WHY DO WE GET SLEEPY?

Have you ever tried to stay awake for a really long time, far later than you would normally go to bed? Luckily I no longer have to work night shift, but in my first few years as a doctor, I had the horribly unnatural experience of forcing myself to stay awake when all I wanted to do was sleep.

By the end of the day, most of us are tired. This biological need for sleep is called sleep pressure. For most of us, when we get up in the morning, we are alert, rested and completely unable to go back to sleep. One substance that builds up in the brain fluid while we are awake is adenosine, which is a by-product of the brain cells accessing energy from glucose. Higher levels of adenosine increase the drive for sleep. Interestingly, caffeine blocks the receptors for adenosine, which is why it helps us stay awake (and why so many shift workers are addicted to coffee!).

Our bodies also have an internal clock, called a circadian clock. At the same time each evening, a gland in our brain called the pineal gland releases melatonin, which also helps induce sleep. This is influenced by light and by ambient temperature.

While we still don't know all the reasons we fall asleep, sleep must be incredibly important for survival, because almost every animal seems to do it. Every animal takes time away from finding food, reproducing and looking for predators to enter a state of decreased consciousness. If you are feeling the need to sleep, don't fight it!

11

CHALLENGING YOUR BRAIN

Although education gives people a higher baseline, it is the activities we keep doing that can slow the rate of cognitive decline.

The majority of people reading this won't get dementia. How do I know this very reassuring fact? Because population studies show that most people reach old age with their cognition intact. Yes, our brains do work a little differently with older age, but this doesn't take away our capacity to learn. Just like a muscle, we can challenge our brains to strengthen neural connections.

The domains of brain function

When I see a patient who is worried about their memory (or, more commonly, is brought in by a worried loved one), after taking a history, I do cognitive assessments with them across a range of brain functions.

Executive function

Executive function is centred in the brain's large frontal lobes and allows us to plan, problem solve and to carefully consider others' points of view. Executive function is negatively affected by sleep loss, stress and physical inactivity, which means that there are many lifestyle steps that can improve its function.

Memory

Memory is of one of the main things that people worry about with older age. The two main types of memory are declarative and non-declarative memory. This is summarised really well in an article published in the journal *Clinics in Geriatric Medicine*:

'Declarative (explicit) memory is conscious recollection of facts and events. Two types of declarative memory include semantic memory and episodic memory. Semantic memory involves fund of information, language usage, and practical knowledge, for example, knowing the meaning of words. Episodic memory (also known as autobiographical memory) is memory for personally experienced events that occur at a specific place and time. It can be measured by memory of stories, word lists, or figures.'

Non-declarative memory involves things we know how to do, like singing 'Happy Birthday' or riding a bike. This type of memory remains stable through life, although it can be impacted late in dementia.

Even when we are having difficulty remembering things we just learnt, the brain still responds to cueing, so we can use reminders to help our memory work as well as possible. I do have patients with mild cognitive impairment (see chapter 11) who are able to compensate well for their memory loss by relying on a calendar or lists. (I do wonder if memory isn't necessarily worse with age, it's just that we have gathered so much information that there is a little more to wade through!)

Language

Language involves the ability to find the right words to construct a meaningful sentence. Although we may have trouble finding the right word every now and then, vocabulary remains stable and may even improve over time.

Visuospatial ability

This refers to the ability to physically find our way around our environment. It is the map we carry of the world in our heads, the ability to read a map and relate it to streets around us, or the way we can stumble through our own house in the dark, knowing where the bathroom is. It requires us to hold in our heads a 'map' of the world around us. This remains intact throughout age.

ISSUES WITH STUDIES OF COGNITIVE FUNCTION

A challenge in interpreting cognitive changes with age is that many of the studies are cross-sectional, which means they examine a group of people at one point in time. This can be problematic given how rapidly our world is changing. Many people who are now in their eighties and nineties left school when they were in their mid-teens because they were expected to earn money for their families, often in manual jobs, which is a very different life course compared to today, when far more people are able to access higher education. Another challenge is that in longitudinal studies, which follow people for many years, the people most likely to drop out are those who are the sickest, meaning there is a bias to well survivors. It is also possible that studies of normal ageing include people who do have early, undiagnosed dementia. All of these factors mean that we are a way off definitively answering the question of what normal age-related cognitive change actually is.

If memory loss has increased to the point where it is interfering with everyday life, it's time to get assessed by a doctor (see chapter 15 on dementia).

Retirement from work and cognitive decline

Stepping into retirement is a huge change in life. Even if it has been highly anticipated, it can come with challenges. It is incredibly important to have strategies to keep your brain occupied. For most of us, work provides constant mental challenges, such as learning new systems and processes and solving daily problems. Work also provides an automatic social group – simply by turning up each day we have meaningful interactions with others.

Worryingly, there is evidence that retirement can accelerate the rate of cognitive decline. Retirement is associated with a decline in cognitive function. A systematic review published in the journal *BMC Geriatrics* found that post-retirement cognitive decline was greater for people who had been doing more cognitively complex jobs, particularly with other people, which fits with the 'use it or lose it' theory.

However, sometimes the decline may be related to job stress more than the absence of the job. One study included in the review found that people who had higher levels of job strain had a higher rate of cognitive decline. When we are stressed, our brains don't work as well, and we tend to revert to more basic approaches to problems, so if you are continuing to work, it is important to have a job that provides challenge and engagement, not stress.

It is likely that a key strategy to maintain or even improve your memory and thinking is to take on challenging roles in retirement. We are still far from a consensus on the effect of retirement on cognition, and some studies have actually found a positive effect.

It is possible that in these observational studies we are seeing the healthy worker effect, where people keep working because they can, while those with poor health or early undiagnosed dementia are the ones retiring.

MARIKA'S STORY

When Marika retired, she went to a job website and searched under volunteer activities. The first thing she tried was giving directions at the local zoo, but it wasn't satisfying and there was a surprising amount of politics, making it more stressful than it needed to be. Marika had also joined a local adult education group, and since she had skill in working with computers, they asked her to join the committee. This was a much better fit for her, because it allowed her to use and enhance the skills she had. Marika has enjoyed the challenge of the constant need to learn new things, and the collaborative and supportive environment of the group. Her responsibilities have ranged from bringing in an online payment system, to planning the roster for speakers. Marika says that she has been able to cope because she is very comfortable asking for help. In addition, she has intermittently taken short-term contracts for paid work, just so she knows she can still do it.

Marika has picked up on the key strategies for maintaining our brain's ability to learn and use information: daily practice. Even socialising has a powerful impact, not only because it feels good, but also because sharing ideas with people actually uses a lot of our brainpower.

Brain connections

The human brain is the most spectacular instrument for learning and creating that we know of. One of the things that differentiates the human brain from a computer is its ability to synthesise information and to form new connections. Our different brain regions don't work in isolation. An evocative smell can bring back a powerful memory, like a familiar perfume that reminds you of a loved one. Abstract thinking is really our species superpower. This is the way we can make connections between seemingly disparate pieces of information to form a category, or even a new idea. We can apply things we already know to a new situation by making associations. Abstract thinking means thinking beyond what we can see; rather than seeing a dog and only being able to think about that dog, it means being able to think about dogs in general.

Neurons, the cells in the brain, have little tentacles (called dendrites, found near the cell nucleus and axons on the tail) that connect to the neurons around them. The connections between cells are called synapses. When an electrical impulse spreads through a neuron and reaches the end of the tentacle, this releases chemical messengers, called neurotransmitters, that diffuse across the short distance between cells to set off an electrical impulse in the next cell. Basically, this is how one neuron communicates with its neighbour. The more this happens, the stronger the connection between the cells. Each neuron can have *thousands* of links with other neurons, like branches on a tree, meaning there are around 100 trillion synapses. Interestingly, the number of connections isn't as important as how functional and strong they are. We actually have our peak number of synapses at the age of three, which for anyone who has spent time with a threenager probably makes a lot of sense. Growing through childhood and into adulthood means pruning some connections and strengthening others.

For a long time, researchers thought that a mature human brain could not grow new cells, but now they are not so sure. Some researchers believe that the hippocampus can continue to generate new neurons into adulthood, although this is still controversial.

Regardless, we know that older adults are still able to learn.

Improving your brain function

Since our brains retain the ability to learn for our entire lives, it is always possible to introduce strategies to improve brain function. There is a lot of emphasis on brain training and crosswords, but our lives are full of opportunities to challenge our brains.

Meditation

One way to maintain your brain function in older age is meditation. By quietening the mind, meditation can improve attention, working memory and executive function. It also improves emotional regulation, which means better wellbeing.

Meditation is essentially the practice of focused attention. It can be as simple as focusing on breathing in and out, repeating a mantra, or thinking of a particular object. Mindfulness is one kind of meditation. It means being present with your thoughts in a non-judgemental way. (See page 61 for more on mindfulness.)

Research has shown that meditation can even change the structure of the brain. A study published in 2014 compared the volume of 'grey matter' (the number of cell bodies) in the brains of people in middle age who practised meditation with those who didn't.

Although there was a decline in both groups, it was significantly less in those who meditated.

Meditation also lowers the physiological effects of stress on the body, reducing the activity of the HPA axis (see page 52) and decreasing baseline levels of inflammation. These changes are likely to explain the brain tissue preserving effects of meditation.

We are still a way off confirming whether meditation decreases the risk of dementia, but it is certainly something that has benefits in the short-term, and that could improve brain function by reducing stress and improving concentration. If you think that meditation might be something that you would like to try, there are many in-person and online courses available, as well as apps like Headspace. If sitting still isn't your thing, there is also walking meditation or even yoga. It's all about finding what works for you.

ISSUES WITH STUDIES OF THE EFFECTS OF MEDITATION

One limitation of meditation research is that many of the studies are cross-sectional, or only look at one point in time. Another arises when researchers are recruiting people who have meditated for a long time (say 20 years or more) to compare them to non-meditators. People who are already able to maintain this consistent meditation might also have certain personality traits, such as being calm and focused, as well as a fairly organised life. This is called selection bias.

Brain 'training'

You've probably heard about brain training computer programs and apps purported to improve working memory. The idea is that brain training will translate into gains in everyday function to help fight off dementia. However, while some of the original trials looked positive, further studies did not replicate those results.

In one of the larger studies, 11,000 participants undertook six weeks of brain training with commercially available programs. The participants had a battery of cognitive tests at the start, then undertook progressively more difficult training for at least ten minutes three times a week. They were divided into three groups and randomly assigned to either exercises that focused on different areas of brain function or to a sham program. Although all of the participants got better at their assigned training tasks, this did not translate to improvements in general cognitive function.

A challenge of these studies is deciding whether they are measuring relevant outcomes. Most of us aren't too fussed about scoring a few more points on an IQ test, but care deeply about being able to maintain friendships and organise our finances, all of which are cognitive challenges that matter in day-to-day life.

In one of the earlier trials, 2800 people aged 65 and older who were cognitively intact and functionally independent were recruited. Half were randomised to ten sessions of an in-person cognitive training task and half were not. This intervention took place at the start of the trial and was not repeated. The intervention groups were followed for ten years, and even at this late stage, showed improved function in activities of daily life. An important limitation of this study is that less than half of the original participants were still involved at ten years. Many of the original participants had died, so by definition, those remaining were healthier. This study also lacked an active control group, which is important as it is possible that the social benefits of the intervention were the true cause of the improvement.

A 2018 study of people with mild cognitive impairment (a condition that confers a higher risk for the development of dementia), however, showed that brain training could have positive outcomes. The participants were randomly assigned to three groups of 49. The first group received training in memory retrieval strategies, the second were given a psychosocial intervention and the third had no contact or advice about memory strategies at all. The group given memory training strategies showed sustained improvement, even after the end of the trial, and were also able to use these strategies in everyday life. It will be interesting to see if this translates to lower rates of conversion to dementia in the years ahead.

One important factor to look at in these studies is that the time spent in brain training was quite small (often only around ten hours over a few months). Compare this to doing a busy job with constant new challenges, responding to other team members and clients who might have different priorities, as well as forming new social connections, and some time tapping on an iPad seems a little bereft. Keeping our minds sharp needs to be incorporated into everyday life. I frequently see patients who do little with their time but watch TV. Needless to say, when a challenge arises they can't step up. Doing an hour a day of 'brain training' won't cancel out doing nothing challenging for the rest of the day. Doing things that tax our brains is hard, but the opportunities for cognitive enrichment are all around us.

IRENE'S STORY

I heard about Irene from an acquaintance. She was not a patient of mine, but her story reflects strategies I use in my clinical practice.

When Irene was in her mid-sixties, she became concerned about her forgetfulness, and how difficult it was for her to remember instructions. Her teenage grandchildren had become so frustrated trying to teach her how to operate her smartphone that they had stopped trying. Irene had retired at 60, after working as an office assistant for 40 years, and hoped that her memory issues were a combination of her age and lack of mental stimulation.

Irene's GP had her complete a brief test that included drawing a clock face and showing the time, remembering a short list of items, and counting backwards from 100. The results showed that Irene had moderate cognitive impairment and a high risk of developing dementia.

Irene did some of her own research and refused to accept the bleak prognosis. She began exercising daily – riding her bike for at least 30 minutes and if that wasn't possible, doing an exercise class in her home with an online instructor. She also attended a weekly computer class for seniors for several years and set herself daily technology-related goals. For example, scanning and filing old photographs, watching a TV show on her smartphone (this was before smart TVs) and working out the operating instructions for new household gadgets. Irene was incredibly determined. Sometimes it would take her a whole day to work out a new procedure, but each time she succeeded, she felt stronger and more positive. It's now eighteen years since the doctor told her to expect the worst. Despite several chronic illnesses (lung cancer, macular degeneration and heart disease) she is still driving to visit friends and family, enjoys gardening and listening to her favourite science podcasts, and is able to live the life she wants.

Cognitive reserve

Cognitive reserve is the ability to maintain normal cognitive processes, even in the presence of dementia. Cognitive decline isn't always in line with the degree of pathology or changes in the tissues of the brain – the amount of time we have spent in our lives doing things that challenge our brains also makes a difference.

One of the bigger societal shifts we have seen over the last 50 years is that more people are staying at school for longer. This higher level of education seems to be one of the key reasons dementia rates are falling. Doing a mentally engaging job is another factor linked with lower levels of cognitive decline. The reason this works is by improving brain plasticity: the ability to learn and use information.

While higher levels of education are helpful, the effects of occupation and engaging in cognitively challenging activities remains powerful. Even for people in their seventies and beyond, activities that require learning and complex thought are likely to keep these processes strong. Not surprisingly, although education gives people a higher baseline, it is the activities we keep doing that can slow the rate of cognitive decline.

So what are these 'cognitive activities' that are so powerful? Simple everyday things such as reading, socialising, playing music, using the computer or doing crosswords and Sudoku puzzles. The key is finding something that is both challenging and enjoyable, so that you will want to make it part of your everyday life.

Dr Alex Bahar-Fuchs is a neuropsychologist who researches brain training. He says that for brain training to be effective, it needs to be consistent and it needs to keep getting incrementally harder. One problem with group studies is that they don't tell us much about individuals. An ideal training program would be tailored to work on individual strengths and weaknesses to improve cognitive adaptability. He also stresses that any cognitive intervention needs to be looked at in the context of other aspects of wellbeing, including adequate sleep and good nutrition.

BERNADETTE'S STORY

Bernadette came to see me because she was worried about her memory. She had been relying more and more heavily on her calendar and was upset because she had recently missed an important appointment that was on a different day to usual. After speaking to Bernadette, taking a collaborative history from her daughter, and conducting some cognitive tests, I was confident that she didn't have dementia, but this didn't mean that we didn't need to look carefully at her symptoms.

Bernadette had subjective memory loss, a feeling that her brain was not working as well as it could be, and this was distressing to her. Although she was still able to do all she needed to do to function in life, she knew her memory could be better. The questions I ask when I see someone with memory problems go beyond just what they are forgetting. Bernadette was also having significant difficulty with insomnia. She was falling asleep, then waking early in the morning, unable to return to sleep. This was fuelling anxiety, and she would lie in bed at night with intrusive worries, which also plagued her throughout the day.

Anxiety and depression are mimickers of dementia, because they negatively impact the ability to focus and remember. As discussed in chapter 10, chronic sleep deprivation also means our brains are not working at capacity.

Bernadette and I discussed a treatment plan for her anxiety and depression that involved optimising her sleep and seeing a psychologist for this, as well as her anxiety. I also encouraged Bernadette to start undertaking some group exercise classes, both to learn new skills and to have some more social time.

It took time, but with these changes, Bernadette's anxiety and sleep improved, and she found her memory improving too.

Exercise

As we saw in chapter 9, some of the most powerful evidence for improving brain function comes from research into the effects of physical activity. I will always strongly encourage my patients to start doing some regular exercise if they are interested in maintaining cognitive health.

Curiosity and creativity

There are so many wonderful, empowering voices showing us that it is possible to stay cognitively active and engaged into what was once considered very old age. There are scientists, doctors, writers and actors who are recognised as being at the top of their field into their eighties. While some cognitive abilities can slow down with age, there are unique advantages to having lived for decades. As Margaret Atwood said, 'I am the age I am and that gives you a certain advantage too, because I remember a lot of things.'

My patients who are in their nineties and beyond and still have their full faculties tell me that one of the most important things is to remain curious and open to learning. Having the right attitude to trying new experiences is one of the most important steps we can take to stay engaged in life.

12

CONNECTION

Friends help buffer the ups and downs of life.

Sharing an experience with another person is emotionally rewarding. Even if it's something that doesn't require active participation, such as watching a movie, doing it with someone else still feels better than doing it alone. MRI, or magnetic resonance imaging, utilises a magnet to give the most detailed images of brain tissue. Researchers are also able to perform functional MRI (fMRI), which measures changes in blood flow, to determine which parts of the brain are most active when someone is thinking about something, or performing an activity. Of course, since the person being studied is lying in a small tunnel, the range of activities is quite limited! In a study of pairs of friends, researchers put the friends in fMRIs in adjacent rooms and told some they were viewing the same images as their friend, and some were not. Those who believed they were sharing the experience with a friend found it subjectively more enjoyable, and had more activity in the reward pathways in the brain. These findings are telling us something we instinctively know: friendship feels good.

Early humans started using fire around one million years ago, although this is hotly debated. While our own species, homo sapiens, now dominates the world, we are still physically weak and fragile compared to most others. For most of human history, we have relied on hunting and gathering for our food and safety, travelling in numbers to protect us from predators. From an evolutionary perspective, our survival depended on the harmony of the group and the strength of the bonds between its members.

Having the support of friends during times of challenge is wonderful, but it is not just the practical help friends can offer that is beneficial – it's the companionship and connection.

JUDY'S STORY

When Judy got up the courage to leave her emotionally abusive partner after decades, it was an incredibly difficult time for her. Although her adult children knew what had been happening and were very supportive, the belittling and gaslighting she had experienced had made her too ashamed to confide in anyone else.

When I asked Judy how she got through this awful time, she had a one-word answer: 'friends'. When she started confiding in her friends, their kind, non-judgemental support was critical to her coming through this separation and finding her confidence as a single woman.

Judy is part of a group of friends who meet for coffee a few times a week. This simple act of sharing time together each week has been enough to develop deep emotional bonds and is something that all the women find incredibly rewarding. They have shared profound events such as the birth of children and grandchildren, supported each other through hardships and had so many laughs along the way.

The scourge of loneliness

One of the worrying consequences from the social distancing essential to stop the spread of COVID-19 is that older people who are already struggling to connect became even more lonely. This in itself has very real health risks.

Studies have shown that people with the fewest social connections have around twice the risk of dying as those with the most connections. What is striking is that this still holds true even when other risk factors, including blood pressure, smoking and diabetes, are accounted for.

People who are lonely have a stronger psychological and physical reaction to stress; even everyday activities can be experienced as stressful. Researchers recruited 134 healthy adults and measured levels of loneliness using a questionnaire. Participants were given a stressful task of public speaking without preparation and had blood taken to measure levels of inflammatory cytokines before and after the stress. People who reported loneliness had higher levels of inflammation after the stressful experience. Loneliness seems to be an inflammatory state, a key factor in the development of chronic disease.

Loneliness even impacts sleep. This is because feeling lonely triggers stress hormones, making us hyper-alert and unable to truly relax. This could be a throwback to our hunter-gatherer days when being alone meant there was no one to share the load of watching out for the animals that preyed on humans. Our brains remain relatively vigilant, keeping us away from the deep and refreshing sleep we need.

To summarise the extensive scientific literature, loneliness is really bad for you: it activates cortisol-based stress systems and increases inflammation. Loneliness also breeds loneliness: people on the social periphery become hyperaware of potential threats, which leaves them more suspicious of people who might be a potential friend.

The difference between loneliness and solitude

One of the most interesting things about loneliness is that it is a subjective experience. People can be surrounded by others, yet still feel lonely. Some of the loneliest people I have met are married.

Recently I met Janine, who is caring for her husband who has dementia. Even though they are always together, Janine is profoundly lonely. Her husband no longer consistently knows who she is, but he certainly knows if she is not there. He is paranoid and suspicious of others coming into the house, including their daughter. Although Janine still loves her husband, he is not able to give her the intellectual companionship and emotional support that he could earlier in their marriage. And she has been left isolated from all of the relationships that can sustain and support her, including those with friends, extended family and even their children.

Janine loves her husband and looks after him out of love, but it is certainly having an impact on her own health. Janine has considered that in the future he might need residential care, but at this time, she wants to continue to be his carer.

Conversely, some people are very happy with their own company: they don't feel that their life is lacking if they are on their own. These people are alone, but not lonely. What matters is whether you are happy with your social circle, not how it measures up to others.

As any of us would attest after a lovely meal with friends, being social can make you feel better, but what particular types of social activity have the most impact on us as we age?

Firstly, it needs to be a social situation where we feel we are actively participating. It is entirely possible to be part of a large group of people without knowing who any of them are, and to feel too nervous to strike up a conversation. This means that having a coffee with one friend is more socially satisfying than sitting in a lecture theatre with dozens of strangers and not speaking.

Secondly, it needs to make us feel nourished and energised. If you come away from spending time with people feeling emotionally drained (say, after a large party where you don't know anyone and have to shout to be heard above the music), this is not exactly beneficial.

The key is to find social experiences that meet your particular needs, whether that be a raucous party or a walk with just one close friend.

The health benefits of being social

For most people, spending time with those we love is incredibly nourishing for our own wellbeing. Not only does it feel wonderful, it also has real physiological benefits.

Socialising helps regulate immune function. People who have satisfying social circles have lower levels of C-reactive protein, an inflammatory marker.

Multiple studies have reported that people who have higher levels of social engagement are less likely to develop dementia. These studies have come from multiple populations in many countries, including the USA, France, Spain and Taiwan. People with higher levels of social engagement perform better on tests of brain function, including memory, abstract thinking and processing speed.

The Midlife in the US study has looked at a cohort of adults aged from their thirties to their eighties who were recruited in the mid-1990s. During the two waves of data collection, researchers measured the frequency and quality of social interactions. When this group had cognitive testing over a decade after the study began, the researchers found that people who had high-quality social connections had better brain function. This applied to people of all ages and ethnicities, and to both men and women. Even people younger than 65 who had higher levels of strain in their relationships had lower scores on memory assessment.

Of course, it is possible that people with better brain function have more rewarding social relationships to begin with, and so there is a bidirectional relationship. Given that this positive relationship starts early in life, it does seem that 'exercising the social muscles' is a way forward for brain health.

I often see large groups of people in cycling gear having coffee together at one of my local cafes after they've been for a ride. This is one of the other benefits of being social: with the right friends, social relationships can also promote healthy behaviours. If you spend time with people who are interested in living well, this can promote being active as a 'normal' behaviour.

The downside of social connections

Of course, relationships can also promote unhealthy behaviours. For example, there is evidence that adolescents who spend time with people who take drugs or smoke are more likely to take these up. In Australian culture, at social events, there is enormous pressure to drink alcohol. Even obesity can be catching.

Negative interactions with friends or family can also be harmful to wellbeing. It is important to reflect on how you feel after you spend time with an individual or group and to assess whether you want to spend more or less time with them. For family, this might mean coming together to speak about issues and finding ways to move forward without conflict.

MARLA'S STORY

Marla, 48, met her husband when she was 20 and they were both at university. He was a couple of years older, sweet and funny. They were both smitten, and a few years later got married. At first they were both working, and progressing their careers, then they decided to have their first child. Because Marla was breastfeeding, it made sense for her to stay home for longer, and she loved having this time with her baby. She had only been back at work for a few months when she became pregnant again. After having the baby, Marla went back to a part-time job. The role involved less responsibility than she'd had previously, but she enjoyed her work, and her family also depended on her income.

When Marla and her husband first married, the housework had been shared reasonably evenly, but while Marla was on leave with the children her husband had worked long hours, so it made sense for her to cook and shop as well as taking on the childcare responsibilities. Somehow, when she returned to work part-time, these things remained her responsibility. If she asked her husband to do something, like tidy up after dinner, he would do it, but the constant strain of having to think of everything that needed to be done, and having to ask her husband to help created an undercurrent of irritation that undermined their bond. Eventually, after 20 years of marriage, they separated.

'Marla' is actually a composite of a few people I know who have told me the same story: their marriage fell apart due to resentment over unequal roles within the household.

Of course, comparing the early days of dating to the daily grind of being married, particularly during that strikingly non-romantic period that involves raising children, is like comparing an Instagram holiday to a trip to the supermarket. Still, plenty of marriages do survive child-rearing and, according to the older people I've spoken to who are still happily married, the secrets are good communication along with shared interests, as well as that all-important sharing of the mental load.

Are married people healthier?

A happy marriage is, without doubt, a source of support and love, and also motivates us to take care of ourselves, which improves our health. However, people who are *unhappily* married actually have poorer health than those who are divorced. This is because constant conflict or feeling lonely in a relationship creates stress that affects our immune system.

The health risk in an unhappy marriage is even starker later in life. This may be because the overall risk of poor health is greater in older age, so as physical resilience is lost, the effects of negative social interactions become more pronounced. This may also be because of an accumulation of stress over a lifetime, but we need more studies to confirm this.

Marriage has historically been better for men's health than women's. This is likely because of the traditional role of women as the carer and household manager. Women take on responsibility for everyone else's health, often at the expense of their own. Men who are married also eat more nutritious foods than unmarried men, and don't tend to drink or smoke as much.

People who are married aren't just healthier because they gain an exercise buddy and healthy eating companion, although these things certainly help. It is often financially beneficial to be married, too. There is also psychological support and a broader and more integrated social network. One of the key aspects of a happy marriage isn't just getting support, it's giving support, which has its own benefits.

Perhaps one of the reasons that men get more benefit from marriage than women is that women have more connected relationships outside the marriage than men do. Social constraints mean many men don't share emotions with anyone other than their partner, where women are more comfortable doing this. If men lose their one and only emotional confidante, they can be left very isolated.

Are people who have children healthier?

As a mother of three children, I can say with authority that having children does not make my life easier. With the level of stress that can come from parenting, particularly for women who lack social and practical supports, parenting small children is not particularly associated with happiness, but this changes in older age.

Some of the challenges of having children can come from the way that our relationships with them change over time – particularly during adolescence, when it is normal for children to push away from their parents. Although this can hurt, it means that you are raising young adults who want to stand on their own two feet.

Positive relationships with adult children can be incredibly good for wellbeing and brain health, even reducing the risk of dementia. Dr Kathy McCoy, author of *Making Peace with Your Adult Children*, explains that we must accept changing roles and realities. As children grow to adulthood and start their own families, the parent is no longer the priority. It is important to celebrate this and to embrace the new people in their lives. Dr McCoy also advises that some emotional distance can be a good thing. Giving your child space to sort out their own problems can actually improve the overall quality of your relationship.

Relationships with grandchildren

There is nothing like a cuddle from a small child. The feeling of their arms and legs wrapped around you and their little head nestled on your shoulder is one I wish I could bottle. Although it's important to have both give and take in social relationships, this one is an exception: the little ones do the taking and we do all the giving, and that is the way it should be – the giving is its own reward.

Caring for grandchildren isn't just a wonderful way to build a relationship, it might actually help you live longer. In a study of 516 Germans aged in their eighties and beyond, those who regularly cared for grandchildren gained five years in life expectancy. Looking after grandchildren combines physical activity, purpose and fun, and these effects have a real biological impact.

For those who provide custodial care of grandchildren, the effects do not seem to be as positive. There is a big difference between having the grandchildren one or two days a week, and being there day and night and assuming financially responsibility for yet another family after you've already raised your own. Data from the Australian Longitudinal Study of Women's Health has shown that women who live with the person they care for are more sedentary and have poorer diets. This is probably because the time spent being the primary carer leaves little time for self-care and increases stress, particularly financial.

Regularly spending time with grandchildren is also beneficial for the children themselves. In a study of adolescents, those who were closer to their grandparents were more resilient to life stress. I suspect that this shows one of the most important aspects of intergenerational relationships: the transfer of knowledge. It is likely that these adolescents were learning from people who have developed a lifetime of wisdom in dealing with life's ups and downs. One of the most powerful parts of our social brain is that we can communicate complex ideas, and so everyone can benefit from the wisdom of age.

Making friends as we age

Our friendships are often based on shared experiences, interests or life stages, and all are important. At certain stages of life it seems much easier to make new friends, such as when we start primary school or university. When our own children start school, we are introduced to a whole new social cohort who are all in the same position – endlessly picking up and dropping off children at school, at sporting and creative activities and at birthday parties. This shared experience means we're very likely to make new friends.

Going further into adulthood, it can be more difficult to make and maintain new friendships, unless we are lucky enough to have work colleagues who also become friends. While friendships usually start with shared interests, it takes a time investment for them to flourish, which can be a challenge with all the commitments of adult life.

This can be compounded with retirement, when those automatic social interactions at work are lost, particularly since so many of us live in households of only a few people. For older adults, becoming unwell and having limited mobility or having a spouse who is unwell are also risk factors for isolation.

Family remains important at all ages, but as we get older, seeing our friends is an incredibly powerful way to cultivate positive emotion. We live in a time with an epidemic of loneliness. We prioritise being independent, but sometimes that can mean forfeiting our emotional connections.

Margaret Manning, founder of the online community Sixty and Me, wrote: 'The fact that you are feeling lonely is not your fault. Nor is it something to be ashamed of. Once you admit this, you are more than half way to building the social life that you deserve. Loneliness is your mind's way of telling you to get out there and engage with the world. The longer you stay in your own cocoon, the greater the chances that you will slip into an even darker mental state, like depression. So, act now!'

Men and loneliness

I recently gave a talk at a local Rotary club. Most of the members were men. The meeting began with a welfare update. Members spoke about who was having medical or life challenges, and how they could support each other. This was incredibly heartening, because social isolation is such a huge problem for older men. In a study in England, 14 per cent of men report social isolation, compared to 11 per cent of women, and 23 per cent report having less than monthly contact with their children, compared to 15 per cent of women. In Australia, men aged 85 and older have the highest age-specific suicide rates. When it comes to forging social connections and sharing feelings, men are often influenced by restrictive social norms. This means that for male isolation to end, attitudes will need a change at the societal level. In the meantime, I hope more men are able to find groups where they can share their joy and sadness and know they will be met with care and support.

Putting yourself out there

If you have made a major life transition such as retirement, separation or a tree change, chances are you will have lost some of your daily social circle. But don't worry – there will be other people out there in exactly the same position.

Social media means that we can maintain connections with old friends we might have drifted away from over the years. There are also online communities for people over 60, such as Sixty and Me (sixtyandme.com) and Over Sixty (oversixty.com.au), where it is possible to get support from people all over the world who are going through similar experiences. There is even an online community called Stitch (stitch.net), which is a site for people over 50 looking to expand their friendship group.

Other options include joining a community group (walking, gardening, cycling etc), becoming a volunteer, or enrolling in an adult education group, all of which offer terrific opportunities to meet new friends.

Putting yourself out there can be daunting, but it feels this way for almost everyone. Chances are, the person standing alone by the coffee station feels just as nervous as you do. Walking over to say hi could be the start of a beautiful friendship.

MAKE FRIENDS A PRIORITY

Teresa Seeman is Professor of Medicine and Epidemiology at the Geffen School of Medicine at UCLA. Professor Seeman has spent decades studying the relationship between social connection and health. Her research has highlighted that social connection has benefits at every age, but can be particularly powerful in our older years. She is 66 and with a father in his nineties, and has no intention of retiring from the work she finds so rewarding.

As an expert on the positive impact of social connection, I asked her how this experience and knowledge shapes her choices. While she is careful about what she eats, and runs half marathons, she says, 'I feel like connecting with friends and family is the most important thing and I prioritise that in ways I didn't when I was younger.'

In a world where busyness is worn as a badge of pride, we really underestimate the importance of spending time with friends.

13

NURTURING WELLBEING

Living a meaningful and satisfying life is an active, not passive process.

In previous chapters I have explored how nutrition, exercise, sleep, cognitive challenge and social connection can help us avoid disease, slow ageing and improve our mental health. However, in the process of making any lifestyle changes, it is important not to lose sight of the real, underlying goal: enjoying life. Part of enjoying life is happiness. It is worth taking a moment to think about what happiness actually is. At a simple level, happiness could be defined as experiencing mostly enjoyable emotions, such as pleasure, pride, joy and interest, with infrequent, but not absent negative emotions, such as boredom and sadness. Someone who describes themselves as happy still experiences the full range of emotions.

Professor Martin Seligman, one of the leaders in the field of positive psychology, defines happiness not only as pleasure, but also as a life with engagement and meaning. Engagement refers to flow, the feeling of being totally absorbed in what you are doing – so much so that other sensations fall away. Meaning refers to doing something that you feel is bigger than yourself. As Aristotle said, 'Happiness is a state of activity.' This refers to the idea that happiness isn't just passive enjoyment, it's found in doing activities that align with your values, participating in life and feeling like you are contributing to the greater good.

This is distinct from pleasure, which involves doing activities we enjoy, but is more superficial and is likely to be short-lived.

We can thank the Ancient Greeks for a more profound definition of happiness, which they called eudemonia (literally 'well spirit'). Rather than feeling good or satisfying appetites, eudemonia is about activities of the soul that align with virtue, which Aristotle elaborated to mean striving to achieve the best that is within us. This is closer to the idea of wellbeing, a concept that combines physical, mental and social health. Wellbeing can mean having enough money to pay the bills, having loving relationships with others, being physically able to engage in life and getting sufficient sleep. These things are all interrelated.

Wellbeing is a very individual concept. It's worth taking some time to think about what it means to you.

Can we measure wellbeing?

Professor Carol Ryff is one of the pioneers in the field of wellbeing research. In 1989 she published a paper called 'Happiness is everything, or is it? Explorations on the meaning of psychological well-being', which has been cited more than 13,000 times. Professor Ryff identified that there was a major gap in the research literature, with no formal way to measure domains of wellbeing. Based on her review of the studies at the time, she identified five domains of wellbeing:

1. **Self-acceptance** – holding a positive view of yourself (in the present, past and future), including making a realistic appraisal of your own strengths and weaknesses.

2. **Positive relations with others** – the ability to have loving, meaningful relationships and being concerned about the welfare of others (see chapter 12).

3. **Autonomy** – being able to self-regulate and to have an internal locus of control, rather than being driven by external social pressures.

4. **Environmental mastery** – being able to manage the world around us and to recognise and utilise opportunities that arise.

5. **Purpose** – being able to work towards goals that are meaningful and important to us.

Professor Ryff developed ways of measuring these five domains using questionnaires; a higher score across these domains means a higher sense of wellbeing. These domains are also areas that we can all reflect on to look objectively at our own wellbeing.

Other measures of wellbeing have looked at life satisfaction, asking people how happy they are overall with their lives. Other scales have looked at hedonic wellbeing, which refers to how often someone experiences certain emotions such as happiness, sadness, anger and stress.

Even the simple question of how people perceive their own health can actually predict survival. In a multi-country study people were asked the simple question 'How do you rate your overall health in the past 30 days?' with response options ranging from 'very good', 'good', 'fair', 'poor' and 'very poor'. After four years, people who had assessed their health as 'poor' had an increased chance of death compared to those who rated their health as moderate, even when accounting for other related factors such as smoking.

It might be that those who rated their health as poor were already getting sick, but self-perceptions of quality of life and health are highly subjective. When I conducted some research in a hospital setting, 67 per cent of people rated their quality of life as good and 58 per cent as good or excellent, even though they were in hospital. Wellbeing and life satisfaction will differ for each person and is entirely subjective. It can also change depending on how someone feels on the day.

How happy are people in older age?

In many countries (but not all), happiness over the life course follows a U shape, with the lowest level of life satisfaction occurring at age 45–54. Bear in mind that this could relate to particular characteristics and social circumstances for the current generation of people in that age group. People in the former Soviet Union and Eastern Europe actually show a reduction in happiness as they get older. Not surprisingly, one of the best predictors of happiness in older age is physical health. People who have a higher number of physical conditions, such as ischaemic heart disease and diabetes, are less happy.

Why is happiness good for health?

It is still not entirely clear whether happiness helps people to live longer. This is because the long-term population studies can't exclude reverse causality, meaning that although they do control for health factors, it is still possible that these people are happier because of better physical health. However, there are some plausible biological explanations for the links between happiness and health. People with positive wellbeing have lower levels of cortisol release throughout the day, as well as lower levels of inflammation and a less active cardiovascular response to stress. People with higher levels of wellbeing might also be more engaged in health behaviours. Two positive characteristics that have been best studied are optimism and purpose.

THE OPTIMISTIC HEART

Optimism is a personality trait that can increase wellbeing, because optimistic people have high levels of self-mastery. Professor Martin Seligman has spent decades researching optimism.

People who are optimists believe that the future holds good events, and that good things are attainable. This positive view of the future can be protective against depression and anxiety. Optimists are more likely to quit smoking after a heart attack, creating a self-fulfilling prophecy by lowering their own risk for the future. Indeed, optimism is highly correlated with heart health.

In one study conducted by The Women's Health Initiative, 100,000 post-menopausal women were recruited to investigate cardiovascular disease and cancer, and how this related to multiple biological and psychological factors. Levels of optimism were measured at baseline. After eleven years, the women in the study with the highest levels of optimism had a 16 per cent lower chance of death compared to pessimists. There were similar findings in the Whitehall cohort of 7942 British civil servants.

Other studies have linked optimism to lower blood

pressure and better blood vessel health, both important markers of cardiovascular health. In a study of 2280 men with an average age of 70 (inappropriately called the Normative Aging Study, since there were no women), optimism was linked to lower levels of atherosclerosis (plaque deposits in blood vessels).

Not surprisingly, given that stroke and cardiovascular disease are both most commonly caused by atherosclerosis, there have been similar findings linking optimism to reduced risk of stroke.

One important caveat to this area of research is that people who were optimists were also more likely to have higher income levels and better baseline health. Perhaps it is easier to look on the bright side when life has been a little kinder. Having said that, there can also be some advantages to having a less optimistic world view – such as being better at assessing risk. Either way, understanding how optimism works could be a step towards improving wellbeing.

A sense of purpose

When I am helping patients make lifestyle changes to improve health, one of the first things I ask is what is important to them. The motivation to make positive changes in health behaviours comes from feeling like our lives actually matter. Having a sense of purpose – a belief that our lives have meaning and that there are goals we are working towards – has a strong impact on physical and cognitive health. This is because a sense of purpose gives meaning to life. Purpose can be measured using a questionnaire. Research suggests that it contributes to reduced overall mortality (particularly stroke and heart attack), as well as decreasing the rate of age-related physical changes and dementia. People with a strong sense of purpose even have better physical function.

One study measured levels of purpose and blood markers for poor health (metabolic, cardiovascular and immune function) for a group of adults aged 25–75 at baseline and again ten years later. People who had a sense of purpose had lower levels of blood markers for poor health. Since greater dysfunction is linked with frailty, this would suggest that a sense of purpose slows the rate of ageing. The researchers also looked at the sense of control this group had over their lives and found that people with a higher sense of purpose had a better sense of control. In other words, they believed that the things they do had a meaningful impact on their lives, which is highly motivating, especially when it comes to exercising or taking your blood pressure medication.

One of the most interesting studies showed that purpose can protect your brain function. A group of people had cognitive assessments during their life, along with a measure of their sense of purpose and then, after death, had a brain autopsy. The findings showed that a stronger sense of purpose protected against cognitive decline, even if people had changes in their brain tissue consistent with dementia.

How do we create wellbeing?

Creating purpose

I firmly believe that enjoying life involves feeling that what you do matters, and that this is important at every age. Finding purpose and meaning isn't always comfortable. Realising any goal requires effort and discipline; put simply, you don't get bigger muscles without doing the exercise.

Living a meaningful and satisfying life is an active, not passive process. It means seeking out opportunities for growth.

One of the challenges in defining purpose and meaning is that we live in a consumerist society where we are constantly urged to buy more things, and that possessions mark success. A high-earning job or a fancy watch are outward, socially constructed markers of success, but might be bereft of meaning for the individual. For example, it is possible to define success as a doctor by dollars earnt, but this can lead to burnout from our emotionally challenging work. For most doctors, our drive comes from the desire to help people, and this sustains us.

Some strategies for developing purpose can come from acceptance and commitment therapy, which focuses on encouraging us to identify what we most value in different areas of our lives. This information is then used as motivation to pursue what is most important to us, even if that means tolerating some discomfort along the way.

We each have our own strengths and resources that we can use to improve our lives and the lives of those around us. Purpose doesn't have to be grand and showy; it can be as simple as volunteering, caring for grandchildren or learning a language. It just means making decisions today based on who you want to be as a person.

A positive attitude to ageing

One of the threats to wellbeing in older age actually comes from negative attitudes towards ageing itself. In a study led by Professor Becca Levy, a cohort of people with an average age of 72 at the time of recruitment were followed for four years. At the beginning of the study, people were given a questionnaire to assess their attitudes towards ageing. After four years, 2.7 per cent of those with a positive attitude to ageing had developed dementia, compared to 6.14 per cent of those who had negative beliefs. This risk reduction also applied to people who were at high genetic risk for Alzheimer's disease.

In another analysis of this cohort, the people with the positive attitudes towards ageing also had lower levels of inflammation and were twice as likely to survive at six years. Self-acceptance in older age might just save your life.

We live in a society that fetishises youth, while people over 60 are seen as past it. Many people have internalised this and as a result, have a negative view of themselves and their future.

This is changing, however, partly because the Baby Boomer generation have never been the type to sit quietly to the side, and they are not about to start now. The youngest baby boomers are now in their mid-fifties, and popular culture is starting to reflect that these people do not see themselves as 'old'. Many of the scientists I interviewed for this book are thought leaders in their field, as well as being past the traditional retirement age.

In a society where anti-ageing bias is still rampant and acceptable, it is worth considering and challenging your own attitudes to ageing. Ageism is a form of discrimination against our future selves. Fear of ageing is often linked to a fear of poor health and dependence. Focusing instead on the positives that come with age, and the fact that most people will enjoy the majority of their later years with health and independence is a good place to start. It's also time we start focusing on the contributions that people of all ages make to society, and to believe that we can do the same.

THE FACE OF AGEING

One confronting aspect of ageing is the change in our appearance. Sagging and wrinkled skin can be a jarring reminder that our bodies are no longer youthful and supple – that we are no longer 'desirable' in terms of socially defined ideals. Each time we look in the mirror, the lines on our face seem to deepen, and instead of seeing them as a beautiful record of all the emotions we have felt in our lives, we often see them as something that should be scrubbed away.

Some people become so distressed by these changes that they try treatments such as botox. However, botox also acts on the nerve receptors in the facial muscles and stops them responding to signals. When we smile or laugh from a place of genuine joy, lines naturally radiate from our eyes. Paralysing the muscles that contribute to this part of the smile will stop these lines from appearing. This may also affect how happy we feel and how well we can interpret others' emotions.

When we are talking to someone, we are also watching their facial expressions, which we unconsciously mimic. This is called embodiment; it's like the mirroring babies do with their mothers. The paralysis of the facial muscles caused by botox impairs our ability to mimic, and so it is harder for others to interpret the subtle nuances in our communication. This diminished emotional experience seems a hefty price for appearing a little younger.

Of course, all the cosmetic procedures in the world are only a superficial solution to the physical effects of ageing. Fillers and botox won't make your muscles stronger, protect your brain or improve the state of your coronary arteries. Ageing is not inherently a bad thing, because it relates to underlying cellular processes. We need to follow the lead of activist Ashton Applewhite and reject anti-ageing bias and the idea that looking older is a bad thing. In fact, it is just evidence of living.

Resilience, reframing and growth

It is incredibly rare to meet someone in older age who has not experienced loss or challenge. I have met people who have had terrible losses, including the loss of a child, and it is a grief that never disappears. Despite this, people do recover, they do go on; they retain the ability to love and manage to find meaning from the most devastating challenges. What I have learnt from people who are coping with grief is that there is no timeline, there is no set period after which grief should be over. People who are navigating loss have identified that social support, a caring GP and keeping busy are all things they have found helpful.

Many older adults actually have high levels of resilience; this is the result of a lifetime of learnt strategies. Psychological resilience refers to a person's ability to adapt well in the face of adversity, trauma, tragedy, threats or significant sources of stress. For older adults, key characteristics associated with resilience are strong community connections, a positive self-view and physical health. It is also possible to develop skills and to learn ways to cope with challenge, which may explain why older women seem to be particularly resilient.

Another attitude that can facilitate successful ageing is developing a growth mindset. The Disrupt Aging movement, started by Jo Ann Jenkins, the CEO of the American Association of Retired Persons, was established to challenge perceptions of what people aged over 50 are capable of. This is a response to the idea that we are incapable of change and learning in older age. The growth mindset is an idea developed by Professor Carol Dweck. She looked at markers of success and identified that people who thought that talents and abilities could be learned, rather than believing that they are innate, were better able to face challenges. This is taught in schools, where children are encouraged to add 'yet'. Rather than saying I am bad at long division, they learn to say I am not good at long division . . . yet. Professor Angela Duckworth wrote about this in her book *Grit*, where she identified that intelligence wasn't the best predictor of success – it was passion and resilience, and that these are characteristics we can cultivate.

ISSUES WITH STUDIES OF PSYCHOLOGICAL WELLBEING

One criticism of psychology research is that many studies have used samples of convenience, which usually means university students who are often studying psychology themselves. Although the physiological findings are fascinating, without replicating them in other groups, we cannot be sure whether they are universally true.

Similarly, we cannot assume that factors that apply in one culture are equally important in another. Some cultures place a premium on individualism, some on the group, so wellbeing factors such as autonomy or positive social interactions may work differently. Even in different stages of life, different factors will be more or less important.

The other issue is replication. For research growth to be considered 'evidence-based truths', other studies using the same methodology must yield the same results. However, it is increasingly recognised in psychological research that many studies cannot be replicated. This means that when another group of researchers use the same methodology, they do not get the same result. Part of this stems from the way we decide whether a finding is statistically significant. Statistical significance occurs when there is a less than 5 per cent chance the result is false – but that still means there is a small chance the result is due to chance alone and doesn't show a true association.

Another issue is the way that science is reported. Journals are more likely to publish positive findings, meaning that studies that do not find an association between two factors are less likely to make it to the scientific record. As a result, the research looks decidedly positive. This is recognised as a problem, and there is a push for all studies to be pre-registered so that negative results are recorded. This would help ensure more negative studies are published and that researchers don't needlessly repeat themselves.

Positive thinking

Shakespeare's Hamlet famously said, 'There is nothing either good or bad, but thinking makes it so.' One of the most effective treatments for chronic pain, insomnia and anxiety is called cognitive behavioural therapy (also discussed on page 141). This is a structured behavioural therapy that involves working with a therapist to identify harmful thinking patterns and reframe them.

As an example, CBT being used to address chronic pain may involve helping the sufferer shift away from the idea that the pain they are experiencing means they are damaging their tissue and reframing it as a more neutral sensation. It can also involve teaching relaxation strategies. Some researchers have looked at the effect of gratitude diaries, where people take a couple of moments each day to write down three things they are grateful for. This can be as simple as the blue sky, a morning coffee and a text message from an old friend. Some small studies have shown that journalling gratitude can even decrease levels of inflammation.

Psychological wellbeing and longevity

Some studies do show a link between improved psychological wellbeing and better health, but not all. There's no guarantee that living with purpose, building resilience and keeping a gratitude journal will make you live longer, but to me, this doesn't matter. Life needs to be enjoyable and meaningful in the present. How can we make choices to improve our future if today is bereft of joy? In earlier chapters I have discussed the way health behaviours such as exercise and diet can improve mental health, giving benefits in the present, not just the future. Life is too short to put off doing projects that are meaningful, or to dwell on things that make you unhappy.

BOB'S RECOVERY

I went to see Bob and his wife in their lovely suburban home, which was a little too large for two 90-year-olds, but was filled with loving memories and ongoing joy. Bob was recovering from pneumonia, which had landed him in hospital. Given his age, it was taking Bob some time to regain full physical function. He and his wife were thrilled to tell me that Bob had been for his first long walk that morning. Bob was a keen participant in his rehabilitation, largely because he had a very important motivator. Throughout their almost

70 years together, he and his wife had gone ballroom dancing almost every week, and he had no intention of stopping. Most of the people I speak to in their eighties and nineties have already achieved the long life most of us are hoping for. They are not generally concerned with how long life will be, but rather, how well they can live it.

POSITIVE PSYCHOSOCIAL FACTORS IN THE HOSPITAL SETTING

In my own research for my PhD, I looked at the impact of positive psychosocial factors for people aged 70 and older who had been admitted to hospital. Being admitted to hospital is a sentinel life event. Many older adults don't recover well, but I wanted to focus on those who do. With the help of my supervisors, Professor Kwang Lim and Professor Ruth Hubbard, I designed a trial to look at whether people with a higher number of health assets, which are protective psychosocial factors, were less likely to be frail. These health assets included having a higher level of education, emotional connection, adequate financial resources, positive self-assessment of their own health and a sense of control over their life. Even though many of these factors related to life decades earlier, people with a higher number of health assets were less likely to be frail.

For people who weren't frail, a higher number of health assets also increased their chance of being alive three months after hospital, but this relationship was lost for those who were most frail. Mechanistically, some of these assets make sense. For example, those with a higher level of education are likely to have a higher level of health literacy and be better able to understand their illness and what they could do for recovery. Others need more research, such as the influence of self-rated health, which has also been shown in numerous other studies.

It is also interesting that for the most frail, a higher number of positive psychosocial factors didn't help. It might be that once someone is extremely frail, there are so many things wrong that these factors no longer have an impact. For me, this research also raises many questions, including what we can do as clinicians to identify protective factors for our patients and help them access and utilise these.

14

MAKING CHANGE

Now is the best time to start living the life you want.

THE BALTIMORE EXPERIENCE CORPS TRIAL

The best place to start improving your health might not be where you think. In a study led by Professor Linda Fried from 2006–2009, a group of older adults signed up to a mentoring program for primary school students at risk of poor academic outcomes. The study was designed to foster social engagement and purpose, but the researchers suspected there might be other effects as well, and they were right.

Each volunteer spent around fifteen hours a week with their assigned student. When the volunteers spent time with the students at school, they weren't just sitting in the classroom: they were going outside with them at play, going to the library and the cafeteria. All of a sudden, without meaning to, they were walking more. Many of these schools had been built over two levels, meaning that the participants were also heading up and down stairs. All this incidental exercise added up, and these people who'd had to pause on the landing at the start of the school year found that they could get all the way to the top without pausing for breath. Some even gave up their walking sticks. This translated to maintenance of good functional status in day-to-day life over the course of two years.

The reason these people signed up to the program had nothing to do with fitness. They just wanted to help children, but in doing so, they improved their own health.

What motivates you?

I don't want you to draw up elaborate diet and exercise plans in order to improve your health. Instead, I would like you to identify things you do that make you feel good about yourself. It might be your ability to grow roses, it might be that you help an older neighbour with their groceries, or that you have started a new exercise class. Here are some questions to help get you started:

- What do you like about yourself?
- What do you do that makes other's lives better?
- When was a time you made a decision you were proud of?
- When did you last learn something new?
- During the past few weeks did you ever feel pleased about having accomplished something?

Your answers to these questions will show you what you value, and where you find purpose and meaning in your life. It will also give you a framework for your health goals.

Set your goals

Reflecting on your own values and motivations, I would like you to set yourself two challenges:

1. Do something for your health every day. This is a smaller, achievable goal. It might be including more vegetables in your evening meal, or getting up and going for a walk every morning. It might even be sticking to a consistent bedtime every night. This needs to be something you can do every day, so that you can feel a sense of progress.
2. Choose a longer-term project. This could be learning a language, participating in a charity walk, finding a volunteer activity, making a family tree or joining a committee at your club. This needs to be something that matters to you, so it needs to fit with your own values.

It is important to try and incorporate something every day because this helps to create habit, which in turn makes it easier to make positive change. It also means that each day it is possible to reflect on what you have achieved. As mentioned previously, most health behaviours will have short-term benefits as well as in the longer term, and I think that this can be very motivating.

Working towards a longer goal is important to develop meaning and purpose. Some of you will already feel like you are very happy with your life. But challenging ourselves, whether mentally, physically or both, is incredibly important to helping us stay well into older age. There are a wide variety of ways to do this. Again, it will come back to your own skills, resources, values, likes and dislikes.

It is also important to reflect on positive emotions. As discussed on page 190, some people will find it very helpful to keep a gratitude journal. While it might seem trite, there is real evidence that doing this can help us train ourselves to focus on the positives.

It is important to start with the psychological aspects (your motivations, your goals and staying positive), because these are the things that will help keep you from falling back into old habits.

Take a holistic approach

Once you have worked out your goals and motivations, it is time to start getting your mind and body into shape. The three foundation stones for doing this are sleep, nutrition and exercise. I realise that it can seem daunting to overhaul three major aspects of your life in one go, but they actually facilitate each other.

For example, let's say your goal is to get more good-quality sleep each night. One way to improve sleep is to exercise more, and to shift your body clock by getting up earlier and getting out in the daylight (this is why a morning walk is a great idea). Not going to bed on a full stomach also improves your sleep, so the next step might be to eat an earlier evening meal and stop after-dinner snacking. Given that our after-dinner snacks tend to be foods like crisps and chocolate, cutting these out has reduced your intake of ultra-processed foods.

If you are eating your evening meal earlier, try to ensure your meal is high in fibre and healthy fats to keep you going until morning. If you are going to bed earlier and having a more refreshing sleep, you are also likely to find that your appetite is better regulated and the cravings for sweets have diminished. As a result, without even meaning to, you are eating a more nutritious diet.

You don't have to make huge life changes all at once. We are setting up a program that will improve life, so the changes need to be sustainable, rather than perfect. You might already be using some of the strategies described in this book, others might not be for you. For example, I think that the science around meditation is compelling, but at this point in my life it is not something I can easily fit in. With three small children, I can barely get a moment to finish a thought, let alone a quiet 20 minutes to meditate!

I do have my own ways of getting away from the rush of interruptions and having a time of concentrated thought, and one of them is writing. I also find exercise, particularly yoga, incredibly useful for this. There is so much focus on how I am holding my body; even simple poses take a large amount of concentration, which is its own form of moving meditation. For me, even walking is an excellent way to clear my head.

Start slowly

You wouldn't try to run a marathon without training. It's the same with any lifestyle change. What we are aiming for is to feel energised, clear-headed and ready to enjoy life. This means starting slowly, and finding something you love.

For example, if you are not in the habit of exercise, it is really important to ease into it. You will need to prepare your body before you attempt intense workouts. While a combination of strength training (with either bodyweight or weights) and aerobic exercise is ideal, it is important to work up to this. The first step for women is to check in with your pelvic floor and core. Even if you don't have symptoms of pelvic floor dysfunction, lifting weights without knowing how to activate your pelvic floor and core can lead to incontinence.

The other key with starting any exercise program is that it should gradually get harder. At first, this might be as simple as choosing to walk further and faster each week. Once you have spent a few weeks working on your back and core, it is time to start some strength training, ideally with a skilled trainer.

It is also important to work on balance. I strongly suggest doing this barefoot, so you can make the most of the balance sensors in your feet. You can start by taking it in turns to bend a knee and lift one leg up at a time. As you get more stable, you can work on lifting the leg up, and then out behind you. You can also practise going from side to side.

It is very hard to keep up the motivation to exercise by yourself, so if possible, go to a class with a friend. Or even better, hire a trainer, which is cheaper between friends, to work on your own particular needs.

A TO-DO LIST FOR JOY

These are the basic principles of living a life with optimal health. They also happen to make you feel good!

- Start a gratitude diary
- Prioritise sleep
- Nourish yourself
- Move every day
- Take steps to manage your stress
- Learn something new
- Spend time with friends and family
- Find your purpose

This list is not exhaustive or overly prescriptive. Each person reading this will have a different need and tolerance for each component. This also needs to be done in ways that are fun. Spending all day with workmates who cause stress may mean you are around others, but these are not positive social interactions!

Remember that you matter

When children are small, their intense physical needs are all-consuming. Then when they are a little older, there are still school pick-ups, sport, music and parties, as well as all the responsibilities of running a household. It is only when their children are young adults that many parents will regain some time for themselves. For those who are not parents, there can be other responsibilities like work or caring for other friends or family members.

Whether you are caring for young children, adult children, your parents or your spouse, I want you to remember that you matter, too. You deserve health. Self-care is choosing to do things that make you feel better. Even if you are caring for someone else, there is nothing selfish about taking some time to improve your wellbeing. You can't pour from an empty glass, and giving all of yourself to others is not sustainable.

Start now

Health is something that we create and enjoy each and every day. It is not something that we reserve for some rainy day in the future. Life ends for every single one of us, and there are no guarantees about what the future holds. That doesn't mean we shouldn't have hopes and goals for the future, but these need to be meaningful now, too. There is no sense waiting for something to change before you start living your best life. Start living life today. As the saying goes, life is what happens while we make other plans.

If there is one message I hope you take from this book it is this: now is the best time to start living the life you want. There is no point living as long as possible if your life isn't enjoyable. The future is too far away and too uncertain; why not give yourself the gift of wellbeing now?

PROJECT THREE SIX TWELVE

I hope that reading this has made you feel motivated to make some positive changes. Project Three Six Twelve is an online exercise and wellbeing course that I have designed with an exercise physiologist. There is a focus on strength training, nutritious and enjoyable food, and understanding lifestyle factors for positive ageing. This is the practical how-to for the information in this book!

PART 3

THE HEALTH CONDITIONS OF AGEING

Harrisons' Principals of Internal Medicine (Volumes 1 and 2) is considered by many to be the ultimate medical textbook. It runs at over 4000 pages and weighs 6 kilograms. There are far too many medical conditions to cover in this book, particularly including the rare and unusual ones. This section focuses on the things that are common, the things that are highest on the list for mortality or for having a negative impact on quality of life. These are also conditions where some or all of the disease process relates to ageing. Knowing about these conditions can help to get treatment fast, as well as understanding why lifestyle strategies are important for prevention.

15

DEMENTIA

Dementia has overtaken cancer as the most feared diagnosis for adults aged in their fifties to seventies.

The tragedy of dementia is that the loss of the person we love can take place over many years. Becoming our partner's carer can change the relationship, especially if their personality changes in challenging ways. Advanced dementia sufferers can forget things that defined them, like their job or the people in their family. Dementia is a disease that can take away the basis of who a person is, as so much of their identity is forgotten. Others can find themselves lost in an unfamiliar world, struggling to know where they are or what they should be doing. This is why it is so important to understand dementia and take whatever steps we can to prevent it.

GRANDPA

I was 27 when my grandpa died of Alzheimer's disease, aged 82. He was probably in his sixties when he started to show signs of short-term memory loss and increasing irritability. We grandkids thought it was funny that he told the same stories over and over, but eventually his memory problems became more serious as they began to affect his daily function.

Grandpa had the classic 'rapid forgetting' seen in Alzheimer's disease, but he also experienced changes in personality, with increased irritability and loss of judgement. There were rare bright moments. When he still knew who I was, during our visits, I could tell him every five minutes that I was studying to be a doctor, and each and every time this new information would surprise and delight him.

My brothers and I were shielded from the worst of it, but one of the most awful things about this disease was seeing a kind, clever, gentle man change into someone who could be aggressive and frightening. Eventually his care needs became too much for my grandmother and he went to live in a residential aged care facility for people with significant behavioural symptoms of dementia.

These facilities are confronting places, and it was my father and aunt who bore the brunt of these visits.

After Grandpa fell and broke his hip, he never walked again. As his dementia progressed, he also became more mellow, and so his physical needs started to outweigh his behavioural needs. He moved to a different residential aged care facility, which was better equipped for his high physical care needs. My dad would visit him and play the piano, bringing a packet of Grandpa's favourite chocolate biscuits. Grandpa would eat one and then, a few minutes later, having completely forgotten he'd had one, happily have another 'first' until the packet was gone.

Over time, the disease affected more and more of his brain function, until he lost his language and couldn't say who we were. I think he still knew us on some level though, because his face would light up when he saw us.

What is dementia?

Dementia occurs when a disease has caused damage to the brain that impacts memory and thinking to the point that it affects everyday function in work or life.

Although dementia can occur in middle age, the prevalence rises sharply with age. Around one in ten people aged over 65 has dementia, and around one in three aged over 85. Dementia is not a normal part of ageing, and most people will not get it, even in advanced old age.

Some of the most positive research news in recent years is that although there are a more people with dementia (which makes sense, as there are more older people overall), the actual proportion of the total population with dementia is falling. On average, your risk of developing dementia is less than your parents' risk at the same age.

Types of dementia

Dementia involves a loss of memory and cognitive abilities that interferes with daily function. It can be caused by many different diseases. The area of the brain that is damaged will determine the symptoms experienced. For example, there is a rare variant of Alzheimer's disease where damage occurs first in the occipital lobe, which is at the back of your brain and interprets vision. The first patient I met with this condition was an art historian who could no longer identify paintings.

Detailed brain imaging, such as an MRI, allows us to see shrinking (atrophy) of parts of the brain, although people can still have Alzheimer's without identifiable changes. In Alzheimer's disease, where memory loss is commonly an early and prominent feature, the hippocampus is often atrophied.

Alzheimer's disease

Alzheimer's disease is the most common cause of dementia, and usually presents with amnesic memory loss, or the inability to form new memories. The classic changes seen under the microscope on autopsy studies are amyloid plaques and tau tangles, which are basically accumulations of abnormal proteins. Highly specialised scans called amyloid PET are able to identify the level of amyloid in the brain, and to see which parts are affected. These are sometimes used for diagnosis, but cannot be used to determine who will get the disease. (See 'What happens to brain cells in Alzheimer's and dementia?' on page 208.) Alzheimer's disease frequently co-exists with vascular dementia.

The majority of cases of Alzheimer's disease are not inherited. There are some rare mutations where an error in a single gene causes Alzheimer's, so there is a strong family history, but these are very rare. These usually present at younger ages, around the forties or fifties. The gene more commonly associated with Alzheimer's is the ApoE4, but even carrying two copies of this gene (one inherited from each parent) is far from a guarantee that the person will develop the disease.

Vascular dementia

Vascular dementia is caused by stroke, where blocked blood vessels lead to the death of brain tissue. Sometimes these strokes are large and cause obvious motor symptoms, such as weakness in the arm or facial muscles, but they can also be undetectably small. If enough of these 'mini strokes' occur, the accumulated damage can affect memory and thinking processes.

This type of dementia usually progresses in jumps as another stroke affects yet another part of the brain.

Lewy body dementia

Lewy body dementia (LBD) is caused by misfolded proteins in the brain, and shares many symptoms with Parkinson's disease. As well as changes in memory and thinking, sufferers will often experience stiffness, tremors and trouble walking. People with Lewy body disease will often have fluctuations in their cognition, even within the same day, and can also have visual hallucinations. Poor sleep is often an early and prominent feature.

LBD is named for the characteristic 'Lewy bodies', also an abnormal clump of proteins. There is significant overlap between LBD and Alzheimer's disease, and the two can be hard to tell apart clinically.

Frontotemporal dementia

Frontotemporal dementia (FTD) affects the frontal and temporal lobes of the brain. It is much rarer than Alzheimer's disease and is more likely to affect people in their fifties to sixties. It can often present with marked language difficulties and personality changes. Some sufferers might have trouble being able to find the words for familiar objects or people; others will become disorganised or apathetic. Some people will be inappropriate, saying the wrong thing in a social setting, while others can be emotionally labile, rapidly switching between laughing and crying.

Around 10–25 per cent of cases of FTD are inherited and caused by a single gene mutation. Like in Alzheimer's, there can be atrophy of parts of the brain visible on MRI, and changes in blood flow on other imaging studies. People with FTD will have abnormal tangles of a protein called tau that normally helps to stabilise the structure of the brain cells.

Alcoholic dementia

Alcohol is toxic to the brain and, over many years of heavy drinking, can do enough damage to cause dementia. People who drink heavily and have poor nutrition are particularly at risk. This type of dementia usually affects the frontal lobes of the brain, impairing executive function, as well as the hippocampus leading to memory impairment.

Other types of dementia

This is far from an exhaustive list of conditions that can cause dementia. Creutzfeldt-Jakob disease, otherwise known as mad cow disease (which can occur spontaneously, be inherited or be caused by eating contaminated meat), causes a rapidly progressive dementia. Dementia can also occur from repeated brain trauma, as seen in boxers and American football players (probably Australian ones as well).

WHAT HAPPENS TO BRAIN CELLS IN ALZHEIMER'S AND DEMENTIA?

The diagnosis of Alzheimer's is based on clinical findings, not on brain biopsy, so what we know about the actual changes in the brain cells of Alzheimer's sufferers comes from autopsy studies. There are two main pathological changes that occur. Neuritic or senile plaques are seen outside the neurons, which are made of clumps of amyloid beta misshapen neuronal processes. There are also 'neufibrillary tangles' inside the cell, where a certain type of structural protein in the neuron gets tangled and clumps.

This can co-occur with amyloid angiopathy – a build-up of amyloid in blood vessels in the brain that makes them more prone to bleeding and scarring in the hippocampus.

For a long time it was thought that the cure for Alzheimer's would come from preventing the build-up of amyloid plaque. There have been around 150 trials of medications that remove amyloid plaques and none have prevented or halted dementia. This may be because once symptoms develop, the brain damage can't be reversed.

It is also possible that the beta amyloid plaques are merely bystanders, and are not actually causing the death of neurons. This is an extremely controversial theory within Alzheimer's disease research. The strongest evidence for the amyloid hypothesis is that some people have inherited a gene that makes amyloid more likely to clump, which causes an inherited form of dementia. Despite this, not all people with high levels of amyloid in their brains will develop dementia, and this is particularly true for older adults. In older adults the degree of damage to blood vessels is more highly correlated with cognitive dysfunction.

Another theory postulates that dementia (including Alzheimer's) may actually be caused by dysregulated glucose metabolism in the brain. Some have suggested that Alzheimer's disease is caused by insulin resistance in the brain, and refer to this as type 3 diabetes (see page 250 for more on insulin resistance). Insulin-like growth factor seems to have a role in brain metabolism and synaptic formation, and there are receptors for this on the hippocampus, which has a key role in memory formation. There is also strong epidemiological evidence that type 2 diabetes and obesity are strongly correlated with dementia.

Some researchers have postulated that Alzheimer's may be caused by the herpes simplex type 1 virus (HSV1), otherwise known as the cold sore virus. This virus is extremely common, with around two thirds of adults being carriers, so many of us have been exposed, even if we have never had a cold sore and never have any symptoms. (Confusingly, HSV1 can also cause genital herpes, while HSV2 causes genital herpes only.) Varicella zoster virus (VZV), which can cause shingles and chicken pox, is another virus in the herpes family.

Once we have been exposed to any virus in the herpes family, it usually remains dormant in our nerve cells, only becoming active if our immune system is compromised. Professor Ruth Itzhaki of Oxford University has theorised that HSV1 might enter brain cells in older adults, leading to dormant infection. This can be reactivated by stress, higher levels of inflammation or a decline in immune function. Epidemiological studies in Taiwan have also provided some compelling evidence that people with either HSV1 or VZV are more likely to develop dementia, and that treating them with anti-viral drugs reduces the risk.

Other theories about the causes of dementia include iron overload, oral bacteria and other immune-related mechanisms.

What we do know is that cardiovascular risk is related to dementia. This means that healthy blood vessels, which allow the brain to get all the energy and oxygen it needs, are critical to maintaining brain function. This isn't just the big blood vessels, it's the small blood vessels as well, some of which, capillaries, are only just wide enough for one red blood cell. On MRI we can see 'white matter hyperintensities', which refers to scarring deep in the brain from chronic poor blood flow. These changes are more common in people with dementia and are associated with an increased risk of stroke. The best predictors for these are age and hypertension. While age isn't modifiable, hypertension, or high blood pressure, certainly is.

Early symptoms of dementia

While we typically think of memory loss as the main symptom of dementia, there are many others that can precede it. The early symptoms are often quite subtle, and when friends and family look back they often realise symptoms started many years before diagnosis.

In general, dementia will present in a way that is slow and progressive. If someone experiences a more rapid change in their cognitive state, there is usually something else going on, and this needs rapid medical assessment.

The symptoms that occur will depend on which part of the brain is affected by the disease process.

Memory loss

Memory loss in dementia typically involves difficulty learning new skills and retaining new information. Often, memory of older events is better preserved, and sufferers can recall things from their childhood even with advanced disease.

When memory loss is a feature of dementia it is more severe and persistent in a way that interferes with life. An example would be repeating the same question multiple times in conversation, or being unable to learn to use a new TV remote.

Although loss of memory is a commonly recognised symptom of dementia, it is possible for other parts of the brain to be affected instead.

Personality changes

Often the earliest signs of dementia can be quite subtle and insidious, and may not relate to memory problems. People may develop apathy, or a loss of drive and initiative to do everyday tasks. Other personality changes can include disinhibition or becoming suspicious or fearful. Some people who were previously mild-mannered may become quite labile in mood and prone to outbursts. People may also develop a persistent low mood or anxiety, which may confound diagnosis, as dementia and mental health disorders frequently co-exist.

Loss of visuospatial abilities

Visuospatial function means being able to identify a visual stimulus and its location. We all have a mental map of the world, as well as of objects around us, so getting lost in familiar areas can be a sign of dementia. A loss of visuospatial function can mean having trouble with depth perception and perceiving contrast. It can also involve loss of the ability to recognise and interpret shapes, which can affect reading. Loss of function in this area can have serious implications for driving.

Trouble with complex tasks

We don't always realise just how many steps there are in something as routine as a shower, and these need to be completed in an orderly way. People with dementia may start to have trouble with complex tasks that they were previously able to do. As an example, a retired accountant may struggle to manage their finances on an Excel spreadsheet. An accomplished cook might no longer be able to complete the steps required to make a lasagne. Some of these activities rely on procedural memory, but they also rely on executive function: being able to focus on a task and to mentally manipulate complex information. A clinical test of this is to draw a clock, because this requires planning of where to place the numbers. Another is the Trails test. This is a two-part test, the first of which involves connecting numbered dots, randomly placed on a page. The second part is to alternate between numbers and letters, which requires both mental flexibility and the ability to maintain two trains of thought simultaneously.

Language difficulties

Early in the course of Alzheimer's disease, as one of the first cognitive changes, sufferers can experience a reduction in available vocabulary, increased use of non-specific words like 'thing' and increased reliance on well-learned phrases. People will sometimes start using word substitutions, or describe an item instead of using its name. For example, instead of the word 'stapler' they might refer to 'the thing that holds paper together'. When this becomes more pronounced, the person may lose words that were very important to them, like a school principal no longer being able to name her job. There are variants of Alzheimer's disease and frontotemporal dementia where loss of the ability to name objects or people is the presenting symptom. One test of language is to show people a complex picture that tells a story and see if they are able to describe it. An even simpler screening test is to show people a series of pictures of words that are known by most people but are not commonly used, such as a rhinoceros or a crown, to see if they can name them.

Impaired judgement

Our frontal lobes are the parts of our brain that give us the ability to plan multi-step tasks and think through potential problems. Poor judgement in tasks that a person could previously do can be a sign of dementia. Another facet of this is a lack of insight, which is why many people with dementia will not actually realise that there is any problem with their memory or behaviour. This can be one of the hardest aspects of caring for someone with the disease – they will be struggling to live at home and relying heavily on support from exhausted carers, yet all the while denying that they need any help at all.

Diagnosing dementia

If someone close to you has worrisome symptoms, it is really important to take them to see a GP. These symptoms can also be caused by other conditions that mimic dementia, such as depression or anxiety. There are also some physical causes, such as vitamin deficiencies or certain medications.

The doctor will start by taking a history of cognitive concerns that may be impacting day-to-day life. They will most likely perform a physical examination, and a cognitive screening test. The most common cognitive screening test is the Mini-Mental State Examination (MMSE), which is scored out of 30. However, the MMSE doesn't adequately test the function of the frontal lobes of the brain. This means that someone with minimal memory impairment but significant difficulty with more complex functions will have a normal score, but they could still have dementia. People who are highly educated tend to get better test scores, and this can mask dementia. Essentially, if the screening test results are normal but you are still worried, it is best to get a referral to see a specialist geriatrician.

The visit to the specialist will involve a more detailed and individual cognitive history, focusing on the person's particular skills and abilities. For example, it may be irrelevant that a 70-year-old professor of biochemistry is not able to cook tiramisu from scratch, but it might be highly relevant for a chef at an Italian restaurant.

The geriatrician will also take a detailed medical history, including a review of all medications, and perform a physical examination. They may also order an MRI to look for evidence of previous small or large strokes, atrophy or other structural abnormalities.

Some people, particularly those who score relatively well on basic cognitive testing yet are describing symptoms, will need assessment with a neuropsychologist – a psychologist trained in specialised cognitive assessment. This is a very detailed test that can take many hours.

Once an alternative diagnosis has been ruled out, a diagnosis of the type of dementia is made on the basis of the reported symptoms and the results of detailed cognitive assessments and brain imaging. As many of the dementia subtypes have significant crossover in their clinical presentation, clinical diagnosis is imperfect. Absolute certainty about the subtype of dementia requires a post-mortem examination of the brain.

When someone is diagnosed with dementia, the 'average' life expectancy is approximately eight to ten years, but the progression of dementia will depend on many different factors. An individual who has a severe period of illness, with admission to hospital, may develop a delirium and not fully recover their previous level of cognitive function. Some people can stabilise for a time. At the most extreme, people become completely dependent on others for all care, including eating, and are unable to speak.

For most people, dementia is a slow progression. Over time, the original symptoms can worsen and more parts of the brain are affected. In end-stage dementia, the parts of the brain that control motor function, including swallowing, are affected, so the person can become malnourished and food can go into the airway and lung. This puts the person at very high risk of pneumonia, which, due to their weakened state, they cannot overcome. Even using artificial feeding with tubes does not improve survival because the saliva can still go into the lungs. In addition, the very act of inserting a long-term feeding tube into the stomach through the abdominal wall is an intrusive surgical procedure with its own dangers.

Providing 24-hour care is beyond most families and for many, there does come a time when their loved one needs to go into residential aged care. The tipping point is usually when the dementia sufferer has high night-time needs, significant incontinence or challenging behaviours, or when they simply can't be left alone for any period of time. This is an incredibly difficult decision, and one that is often made with great sadness.

Treatment for dementia

Although Alzheimer's disease causes 70 per cent of all dementia, we are sadly still far from a cure. Whenever I see a headline about a cure for dementia, I feel a sense of alarm. The sensational headline almost always refers to a study in animals, or a drug in very early development, which will almost certainly not work. In the ten years between 2002 and 2012, just 0.4 per cent of all drug trials were successful, and these were only for symptomatic benefit, and did not modify the disease trajectory.

There are two classes of drugs that can help treat the symptoms of dementia by boosting levels of neurotransmitters in the brain. The first class are called cholinesterase inhibitors, which increase the levels of a neurotransmitter called acetylcholine. This includes donepezil, rivastigmine and galantamine, and in Australia these are approved for mild to moderate dementia. Trials of these medications have shown a small improvement in cognitive function on testing, and subjective improvement from carers for around 50 per cent of people, although around 20 per cent enjoy a more significant improvement. They have not been shown to have a significant effect on prevention of the development of disability, however. These medications can also cause intolerable side effects, including urinary and faecal frequency and abdominal discomfort, which can sometimes improve with a dose reduction. A less common but more significant side effect is to cause a slow heart rate. For this reason, the person will have an ECG before starting the medication.

The other drug approved in Australia is called memantine, which acts on a different neurotransmitter receptor for glutamate. The original randomised trial included people with moderate to severe dementia who had functional limitations, including showering, dressing and toileting. This was shown to have a small effect, although 71 of the original 252 trial participants dropped out, so the results need to be interpreted with caution. No studies have shown benefit for memantine in mild dementia.

Caring for someone with dementia

The behavioural issues that can arise in patients who have dementia can be one of the most distressing things for family members to manage. Just as every individual has a different personality, the experience of dementia is different for every person. This can be influenced by the part of the brain affected, as well as the person's personality and life experiences. For some reason, similar to babies, this challenging behaviour often occurs in the late afternoon, and is referred to as sundowning.

When we lose the ability to remember, we also lose the ability to daydream, or imagine the future. When we are in an uncomfortable situation, whether it is physical discomfort or boredom, we let our mind wander. People with dementia are stuck in the moment, unable to imagine themselves into a more pleasant place. This can be combined with changes in the parts of the brain that regulate behaviour, meaning that they can act impulsively and without inhibition. Some people will call out, or vocalise; others may wander incessantly.

In cases of moderate to severe dementia, people may not be able to verbalise if they are uncomfortable, or even recognise the source of their discomfort. Just as a small child may lash out physically when they feel overwhelmed by their feelings of fear or frustration, some people with dementia may become uncharacteristically aggressive, even towards the carers they depend on.

If someone you love is showing these symptoms, it can be helpful to look for any sources of discomfort. Clinically, we always start with the simple things, like checking for pain, constipation and urine retention. Boredom is another potential source of discomfort. It can be helpful to know what the person with dementia loved to do (we all like to feel a sense of purpose). Some people respond well to doing versions of the activities that previously filled their days.

Residential care for someone with dementia

One of the common referrals I receive is to treat people with challenging behaviours who live in residential care. These behaviours can include wandering into other people's rooms, showing aggression with carers or exhibiting distress. After I have checked for physical discomfort, my next step is to find out more about the person and what they have enjoyed in life. One woman I met had worked as a farmer her whole life, and was struggling with the confines of the residential care facility. She would often become distressed while seeking her long-deceased father. Her level of cognitive impairment meant it wasn't safe for her to be out on walks by herself, but staff found she was much more settled when they took her out for a walk each day. Another man, a retired engineer, would settle with adult colouring books. Some people, usually women, who have often been incredibly busy their whole lives, will respond well to being able to help with tasks like folding towels. Many people also respond to dolls. It can be incredibly beautiful to see an older woman transported right back to being a new mother.

While sometimes medication can be used to alleviate extreme distress in the context of dementia, the first line is almost always to trial behavioural strategies.

Support for dementia carers

When I see my patients with dementia, I frequently also see an overwhelmed, exhausted partner, son or daughter who is doing their absolute best to help them.

Caring for someone is a marathon, not a sprint. It is a marathon that can have funny and happy moments, but it can also be accompanied by grief. When someone we love needs our help, we want to give it to them, but if we don't fill our own buckets, we put our own health at risk.

If you are caring for someone with dementia, it is incredibly important to take care of yourself and to get help if you need it. Dementia Australia is an organisation with excellent resources for carers. It is also highly likely someone in your wider social circle is going through a similar experience.

It is also important to remember that you can't do the best for the person you love if you are exhausted. Your own physical and mental health needs still matter, and it is not selfish to take some time to do things that make you feel better.

Is dementia preventable?

Encouragingly, rates of dementia seem to be falling. A 2016 study showed that in the USA, the rate fell from 11.6 per cent in people aged 65 and older in a cohort recruited in 2000 to just 8.8 per cent in a cohort recruited in 2012. There are similar findings in the UK.

While more research is needed to clarify exactly why we are seeing this trend, one factor could be higher levels of education. Having a stronger baseline brain function seems to prevent, or at least delay, dementia onset.

A report in *The Lancet* suggests that around 30 per cent of dementia cases could be prevented with regular physical activity, nutrition, education and control of cardiovascular risk factors.

SCREENING FOR DEMENTIA

I can't count the number of times I have sat with the child of a patient with advanced dementia and they have told me how worried they are for their own future. For many people who have cared for a relative with dementia, the stress of seeing someone you love losing themselves is compounded by the fear that this could happen to you. While there are families with an inherited single gene that causes dementia, this is extremely rare.

For every gene, it is possible to inherit different versions, called alleles. There is an allele called APOE4 that is associated with an increased risk of developing Alzheimer's disease. Patients who have two copies of this allele are much more likely, but not absolutely destined, to develop dementia. In addition, almost 40 per cent of patients with Alzheimer's disease do not carry APOE4.

Even for people who have two APOE4 alleles, lifestyle can reduce the risk of dementia. While it is possible to send away a sample of DNA to find out which allele you have, I'd suggest thinking carefully through the implications of having this test. You may find out you have the low-risk allele, but that doesn't mean it's safe to take up smoking, ignore your blood pressure and live off sugary drinks. Conversely, you could have the high-risk allele and spend a lifetime experiencing sickening anxiety every time you misplace your keys.

It is also possible to do highly specialised brain scans that can detect how much amyloid is present, but as we saw earlier, this is not useful if someone already has changes consistent with dementia, as it doesn't tell us about disease severity or prognosis.

In people who are asymptomatic, a higher burden of amyloid plaque is associated with an increased risk of dementia, but many who test positive still won't get the disease. There is also the risk of causing personal distress: if you were perfectly well, would you want to know you were at high risk of developing an untreatable neurological disease? Until we develop good treatments for this disease in the pre-symptomatic stages, screening is not justified.

16

FRAILTY

Frailty is an extremely important concept, because it helps us to understand the physical changes involved with ageing beyond traditional medical diagnoses. It explains why some people don't have 'medical problems' but are just not thriving.

The medical definition of frailty is a loss of 'physiological reserve' that leaves an individual vulnerable to poor recovery from physical and psychological stress.

Take, for example, a urinary tract infection. For most women or men, UTI symptoms will include pain when passing urine, needing to pass urine more often and perhaps a fever. They will go to the doctor and get some antibiotics and will recover in a few days. For older adults who are frail, however, a UTI can cause very different symptoms. They might feel weak and have trouble walking, and in some cases may become confused.

Infection is not the only stressor that can cause this sudden decline in physical function: it could be a fall, a medication change, surgery or a new environment. Importantly, depending on the severity of the decline, a significant proportion will never get back to the same level again.

What we do know is that people who are frail are more likely to develop a new disability, more likely to end up in hospital and more likely to die.

Diagnosing frailty

The concept of frailty as an objectively measurable condition is relatively new, and owes much to the work of Professor Linda Fried. In 2001 she and her colleagues identified five factors in frailty: unintentional weight loss (10 pounds, or 4.5 kg, in the previous year), self-reported exhaustion, weakness (low grip strength), slow walking speed, and low physical activity. Having three out of the five conferred greater risk of adverse outcomes.

One of the major findings of this study was that people could be frail without having other medical diagnoses, such as heart disease, kidney disease or dementia. Some people will just have a degree of muscle weakness and impaired immune function, and it is these people who might develop pneumonia and then struggle to stand.

One limitation of the study is that it did not include people who already had cognitive impairment or neurological disease, so the frailty criteria cannot be applied to them. There are also some challenges in using this measure clinically – for example, if a person can't walk, we can't measure walking speed. Accurate measurement can also be affected by an illness, so it is hard to apply these criteria in the hospital setting.

Professor Ken Rockwood is another researcher whose work has been instrumental in our understanding of frailty. He uses the analogy of the toaster and the aeroplane to explain frailty. If a toaster fails, you've got untoasted bread – no big deal – so toasters are not manufactured with any backup system. However, if an aeroplane fails it is a disaster, so aeroplanes have multiple backup systems to ensure they take off, fly and land safely. While it is still possible for all of these backup systems to fail, the multiple systems mean that this is less likely to happen. Humans are like aeroplanes: we have lots of backup systems, but when we fail it is dramatic.

Older adults who are frail have lost their backup systems. This means that when they have some sort of stress, like an illness, there is a whole system failure. For a person who is at the limits of their physical capacity every day, having something else to cope with can take more strength than they have.

HELEN'S STORY

As medicine becomes increasingly specialised, it is increasingly important to have a team of specialists working together to ensure patients receive optimal management. Most hospitals now have an orthogeriatrics department, where a geriatrician and orthopaedic surgeon come together in their complementary roles to provide care for older adults with fractures.

I was working on one of these units when I met Helen in the emergency department. She was a thin lady in a hospital gown, lying very still with one of her legs slightly shorter than the other and her foot facing unnaturally outwards: the classic presentation of a fractured neck of femur. She was deaf, so I had to communicate through her daughter, Wendy. Helen was 92 and had been living alone. She had enjoyed excellent health for most of her life, and was only on two medications, but Wendy had noticed that in the last few months, Helen had been struggling a bit more than usual. Her appetite had decreased and she had lost some weight, and she seemed to be getting a bit forgetful. Wendy had been visiting daily to check on her mother, and on one of these visits she found Helen on the floor of her bedroom, her fall alarm sitting uselessly on her bedside table.

Wendy called an ambulance and they transported Helen to hospital. Having lain on the floor for a few hours, Helen was already dehydrated by the time she got to hospital, and kept asking where she was. Along with the dehydration, the pain, the pain medication, and the bewildering emergency department, where it is hard to sleep, Helen had many risk factors for developing a delirium, or sudden onset of confusion.

We would generally avoid the physiological stress of surgery for someone in Helen's position, but a fractured neck of femur is extremely painful if it isn't repaired, and without surgical repair, there is no hope of walking again.

Helen got through her operation, but by the evening of the second day she was very confused and had developed delirium, a common complication of hospital admission for older adults. The delirium made her very sleepy, so it was hard for the physiotherapists to get her out of bed. Lying in bed meant Helen was unable to properly expand her lungs and clear secretions, so she then developed pneumonia, which meant yet more days that she was too unwell to do physiotherapy. Although she survived and went to rehabilitation, her memory and walking never fully recovered. After almost two months in hospital she was discharged to a nursing home, where she died a few months later.

What causes frailty?

Ageing is the greatest risk factor for cancer, dementia, heart disease, diabetes, kidney disease and lung disease and these, in turn, are all linked with frailty. However, the relationship only works in one direction: people who have heart disease are more likely to become frail, but people who are frail are not more likely to develop heart disease.

Some people reach very old age with no medical diagnoses. These people are often very healthy, and living a life we aspire to. Because I often work in hospitals, I tend to meet people when things are not going so well. People who reach their late nineties and beyond often don't have many 'diseases' and are on few medications, but they can still be floored by a simple infection; they are still frail.

Frailty and cellular ageing

We know that frailty is connected to age, so it makes sense that frailty is related to cellular ageing, but this has been surprisingly hard to prove. Although we know that the number of senescent cells increases with age, this isn't quite the smoking gun we need to prove causation. (Senescent cells, as we saw in chapter 2, are cells that have been damaged and are no longer able to replicate, but still influence the cells around them.)

One study published in 2018 demonstrated a tantalising mechanistic link between senescence and frailty. The researchers took senescent cells from old mice and placed them in young mice. The senescent cells took hold in the young mice and started to affect the cells around them, leading to even more senescent cells. The researchers then found that these mice had reduced grip strength and walking speed; changes consistent with how we identify frailty in humans.

The researchers also created metabolic stress in some of the mice by feeding them a junk food diet, which sped up the development of frailty even further. Of course, there are the usual reservations in applying the results of animal studies to human beings, but this does at least suggest that senescent cells have an important role in frailty.

It is also likely that changes in mitochondrial function and gene expression (which means that cells can't use energy as efficiently) partly drive the development of frailty. Given that unexplained weight loss and loss of muscle tissue go together, it seems highly likely that this is an important part of why we become frail.

Frailty and inflammation

While we don't yet have clinical tools for measuring cellular senescence or mitochondrial function, we can measure inflammation. People who are frail tend to have higher baseline levels of immune activation, but a reduced ability to respond to an infection. We know this from studies of vaccine response: although frail older adults still respond to vaccines, the response is not as robust. This is why older adults need boosters of some vaccines (such as chicken pox to prevent shingles), as well as receiving more potent vaccines for flu.

Although frailty is associated with higher levels of inflammation, working out what comes first is challenging. Some people have theorised that frailty drives higher levels of inflammation, not the other way around. Hopefully with some more research we will be able to answer this question in the future.

The social determinants of frailty

Working in clinical medicine means I am constantly diagnosing and treating conditions that are related to problems beyond my capacity in a clinical appointment. One of these factors is often socio-economic status. Insecure or low-paid employment, worries about rent and food, and unstable or abusive relationships are all stressful and can all increase cortisol.

There is evidence of a link between stress and frailty; people with higher baseline levels of cortisol are at increased risk of frailty. This makes sense, given that higher cortisol levels are linked with immune dysregulation and metabolic changes.

While many population studies show that people who are financially secure and socially connected enjoy good health, we don't have enough data to understand the specific physiological mechanisms that relate social factors to better health.

It is worth noting that in countries where many people are poor, this relationship is a little different. There are islands in the Mediterranean where people still follow a traditional way of life, growing their own food. These people don't have a lot of money, but they are still among the longest-lived, healthiest people in the world. In their social group, everyone is in a similar financial situation, and they don't have the stress of external pressures and expectations. They eat well, stay physically active and are socially connected, with time for leisure. This shows that it's not being monetarily rich that confers health, it's a combination of lifestyle and stress management.

Coming back to our own society, poverty in older age is one of the biggest threats we face in helping people grow old well. This is particularly true for women, who are far more likely to face financial stress in their later years due to both income inequality and loss of income due to caring responsibilities. Women are less likely to own a home, meaning they face an increasingly unaffordable rental market; indeed, older women are the fastest growing group of homeless. As a civilised society we need to care about our most vulnerable members, and this means agitating for policy change to fight poverty across all age groups.

What happens to people who are frail?

Around 10 per cent of people aged over 65 are frail, and this proportion rises to 50 per cent for those aged over 85. In many cohort studies, almost all adults aged 90 and over are frail.

In large population studies, being frail is associated with an increased risk of death. Although this increased risk is small, and there are many other factors at play, it is still a better predictor than age alone. This fits with what we see around us, with some people remaining fit and well into their late eighties and beyond, while others need help decades earlier.

Frailty isn't just a risk factor for death, it is also a risk factor for losing independence. We forget just how much strength and coordination are required for tasks we take for granted in adulthood. For example, a person who becomes exhausted after walking only a few metres may find it impossible to go to the shops. For those with very weak grip strength and poor balance, showering alone becomes impossible.

Frailty is not the same as disability, but it is a risk factor for developing disability, or for needing help with essential activities of daily living. Disability is a complex area. Some older adults with frailty are very happy to have help – if it is hard to get out, a shopping companion can be very pleasant – but there is no doubt it can restrict quality of life. Slowing the progression of frailty might be one way to delay any loss of independence.

Frailty is not a binary condition (where you either have it or you don't). There are degrees of frailty: someone can be slightly frail and or severely frail, and it is possible to transition between these states.

A fascinating clue to the way frailty can change over time comes from a study of almost 1500 older adults in Beijing. This group was followed for fifteen years and frailty was measured at five, ten and fifteen years. Not surprisingly, most people who were very frail had died by the end of the study period. The outcomes for those who were moderately frail were heavily influenced by protective factors, including financial resources, a happy marriage and a higher level of education. These people had better survival rates and many actually transitioned to a better health status.

Are there treatments for frailty?

The most studied intervention for frailty is exercise. Even for the very frail who live in residential aged care, exercise can improve function. While having a low protein intake and a diet low in micronutrients is a risk factor for frailty, there is still insufficient evidence to recommend particular dietary treatments. In my clinical practice, I do take a dietary history, however, and refer people to a dietician if I have concerns about poor diet.

Frailty is multidimensional and management needs to be individualised. Someone who is mildly frail may still benefit from tight blood pressure control to prevent future heart attacks, but in someone who is more frail, this same treatment might cause them to fall over and suffer a devastating fracture. One of the reasons geriatric medicine developed as a speciality was the evidence that a holistic assessment of medical, nutritional, functional, psychological and social domains is incredibly beneficial to adults in their sixties and beyond. Just as every person has their own skills and strengths to cope with life's challenges, we need to develop lifestyle management plans that utilise these.

A PHYSIOLOGICAL TIPPING POINT

I recently saw a patient who was in her late nineties. The nurses at her care facility were worried that she was depressed because she had lost interest in eating or getting out of bed. When I went to see her, she was surrounded by family and I was struck by the calmness and love in the room. Her family left while I examined her, and I asked her what she wanted. She told me how much she loved her family and how proud she was of her sons, and that she was just tired and wanted to sleep. Although she was fading, she had a deep sense of contentment at a life well lived.

When I spoke to her family afterwards, I told them, 'I think she has decided it's her time.' They said that this was what they were expecting to hear. She died peacefully a few days later.

We used to have a concept of 'dying of old age', which has been lost in the medical model of health. When people become extremely frail they do die of old age in a way, because their bodies become overwhelmed by an infection or other process that they would have been able to fight off in their younger years. We need to remember that this is a natural part of life. There is so much that we can do in medicine to save and prolong life, but knowing when treatment is futile is just as important.

The future of frailty

Frailty is a manifestation of ageing, and is a result of all the influences on a person's life from conception onwards. It provides a holistic overview of health that goes beyond medical diagnoses to look at a person in the context of their everyday life. As more people reach very old age, it is incredibly important that studies of older adults look at frailty as well as the usual chronic diseases. As we have seen in this chapter, someone with a medically defined chronic disease can still be healthy, while someone who doesn't have a condition that meets a medical diagnosis can still be frail.

17

HEART DISEASE

Although heart disease remains one of the biggest killers, it is also one of the biggest medical success stories. Through a combination of preventative medicine strategies and treatments, heart disease survival has improved dramatically.

You probably know someone who has had a heart attack, or you may have heart troubles yourself, but despite its prevalence, there is still a lot of misinformation about what heart disease actually is. In this chapter I want to provide some basic terminology about heart disease and its symptoms.

CHRIS'S STORY

Chris was driving home from her job as a teacher when she noticed that her chest felt tight. She didn't think it was anything serious – after all, she was only 65, very healthy and never smoked – but after a few hours the pain still hadn't gone away and she had started vomiting, so she decided to call an ambulance. The ambulance driver told her it was unlikely to be anything serious, but took her to hospital as a precaution.

When she got to hospital and the doctor looked at her ECG, things escalated quickly. Chris had a serious blockage in one of her arteries and her heart muscle was being starved of blood. The doctor immediately called the cardiologist, who personally wheeled Chris to the angiography laboratory and tried to clear the blockage by feeding a catheter up through an artery from her groin. However, the blockages were too severe to be unblocked in this way.

In denial, Chris's first response was to ask if she could go home. Instead, the next day she had coronary artery bypass surgery, where her sternum was cut open so the blocked blood vessels in her heart could be replaced.

The next few days were awful. Chris had gone from being a fit, active woman to someone who struggled to do anything at all. But Chris was determined to recover. She set herself the challenge of doing a little more each day: first it was one more lap of the ward, then it was getting to the end of the street, then to a coffee shop. She needed to make a speedy recovery: she had theatre tickets with her granddaughters only a few weeks after the surgery, and she wasn't going to miss the show for the world.

Chris feels that her health scare has given her an extra zest for life – she doesn't believe in putting things off now, and tries to make the most of every day.

The heart

The function of the heart appears deceptively simple, but even after decades of trying, there is still no artificial heart that works as well as the real thing.

The heart is mostly made of smooth muscle, which is structurally different to the muscles that you can consciously control. If you think about how tired your legs get after walking all day, it makes it even more striking that your heart can keep beating for as long as you are alive.

Our bodies have a system of blood vessels (tubes) that carry blood around the body. Arteries are larger vessels that carry blood away from the heart and veins are smaller blood vessels that carry blood back to the heart. The veins all come together, like river tributaries, at the large veins called the superior vena cava and the inferior vena cava, both of which drain into the heart. This blood appears dark because the red blood cells are carrying carbon dioxide, a product of cell energy production.

The blood enters the first chamber, the right atrium, then passes through the tricuspid valve to the right ventricle, which is larger and more muscular and pumps the blood into the lungs via the pulmonary artery. In the lungs the red blood cells divulge their carbon dioxide and exchange it for oxygen. The now-oxygenated blood then goes back into the heart, via the left atrium and left ventricle. The left ventricle is the most muscular part of the heart because it sends blood all the way around the body.

Although we think of the heart as an active muscle, to function properly it must be able to both contract *and* relax. Not surprisingly for such an active organ, the heart depends on a rich supply of oxygenated blood being delivered via the coronary arteries. During contraction, nothing gets through, but when the muscle relaxes it allows the arteries to fill with blood.

The coronary arteries branch off the base of the aorta, the big artery that exits the left ventricle to carry oxygenated blood around the body. When these arteries are blocked, either partially or completely, it is called ischaemic heart disease.

Ischaemic heart disease

'Ischaemic' means an inadequate supply of blood. The most dramatic presentation of this is often called a heart attack, which is the result of a sudden blockage of a coronary artery. The underlying cause of this is atherosclerosis, or a build-up of plaque deposits on the inner walls of the artery. Of course, smaller blood vessels can become damaged as well.

The very first stage in the formation of a plaque is called a fatty streak, which is mostly made up of macrophages, a type of immune cell. These immune cells can stimulate an inflammatory response that leads to the thickening of the artery wall and the accumulation of fatty tissue. These plaques can even start developing in childhood and take decades to grow, which is why it is vanishingly rare for a teenager to have coronary heart disease.

The risk starts to increase when people are in their forties and beyond. After many decades, the plaque will have a fibrous cap with a centre that is made up of a fatty core. These plaques can grow slowly over time, gradually blocking an artery. If the growth is slow enough, other arteries will compensate and increase in size to continue the blood supply, although people can still experience symptoms from an inadequate blood supply called angina. A heart attack, or acute myocardial infarction (AMI), occurs when this cap becomes unstable and ruptures. The inside of the plaque is highly thrombogenic, which means it promotes blood clotting, so when the blood is exposed to it, it forms a clot, like a scab, that can block the artery.

The symptoms of a heart attack happen because the heart muscle is being starved of blood. The textbook presentation of a heart attack has always been crushing chest pain. People also use words like tightness, pressure or heaviness. The pain can travel down one or both arms, to the upper abdomen or to the throat and lower jaw. People can also experience shortness of breath, nausea and vomiting, or a subjective feeling of weakness.

When Chris had her heart attack, one of the most sensible things she did was to call an ambulance. Although she was told that her symptoms were not likely to be significant (an experience common to many women), once she got to the hospital she was treated quickly. The cardiologist rushed her to the angiography suite to unblock the artery because time is critical for the survival of cardiac muscle. The sooner you get treatment, the more heart muscle can be saved.

Treatment for heart disease

Although doctors could recognise signs of a heart attack in the mid-1900s, the only available treatments at the time were aspirin (which decreases clotting by decreasing platelet activity in the blood) and bed rest. It wasn't until the 1980s that streptokinase (along with aspirin) were administered to break down the clot and allow blood flow to return to the heart.

In most hospitals streptokinase/aspirin have been superseded by percutaneous coronary intervention (PCI), where a small tube or stent is threaded to the blocked blood vessel in the heart through a vein starting in the groin. Dye that can be seen on radiological imaging identifies the blocked artery, and a metal coil is inserted into the affected artery to restore blood flow. This can dramatically increase the chance of survival.

Sometimes it is impossible to perform PCI because the segment of diseased artery might be too long, or it is a particularly critical blood vessel called the left anterior descending artery. The decision of whether to choose PCI or open bypass surgery is often made after a multidisciplinary meeting between surgeons and cardiologists to determine the best option for the patient. The first successful coronary artery bypass grafting occurred in 1961. These advances in disease treatment and prevention explain why we now enjoy increased survival in adulthood.

But the gains in life expectancy from better management don't just come from treatments in the hospital. Today, when someone leaves hospital after a heart attack they will be carrying a bag of new medications to thin the blood, decrease cholesterol and lower blood pressure. Many people who survive the heart attack will still be left with some damaged heart muscle, leading to the heart pumping less efficiently. This is called heart failure (see page 241 for more about this).

Women and heart attacks

Although women are less likely than men at younger ages to have a heart attack, of those who do, they are more likely to die. Women are also more likely than men to have 'atypical' symptoms (a problematic term because it defines men as the norm), which can mean they delay presentation and their doctors don't recognise that they are having a heart attack. Around 40 per cent of women who have an AMI don't experience chest pain. In a study from the USA, of more than 10,000 people who presented to emergency departments with evidence of acute coronary syndrome, women were more likely than men to be sent home. This was particularly true for women aged under 55. Women are more likely than men to have their symptoms dismissed and less likely to receive certain treatments. Even studies of coronary heart disease mostly recruit men.

In 2017 the American Heart Association released a statement highlighting the need for a better understanding of ischaemic heart disease in women. This is seen as an important area and there is a growth in research in this area.

> ## THE BENEFITS OF BEING TREATED BY A WOMAN
>
> If you are a woman going to an emergency department because you are worried you are having a heart attack, one way to improve your chances of survival is to request a female doctor. In a study from Florida, women who were treated by a female physician had a better chance of survival than those treated by a man. The study's authors hypothesised that this could be because female doctors are more aware of gender differences in the presentation of heart attacks. Male doctors who worked in departments with more female doctors did better at diagnosing and treating women with heart attacks. Just another reason gender equality in medicine is so important!

Heart failure

Not all heart problems are due to ischaemic heart disease. Heart failure is another condition that becomes more common in older age.

Heart failure means that the heart is not able to pump efficiently. It can be poor at relaxation and filling, or poor at contracting and emptying.

As we saw in the previous section, a heart attack that damages muscle can lead to heart failure, but there are many other causes. Heart failure is also linked to diabetes and obesity, where it can be the result of the heart becoming stiff and not filling with blood properly. Other causes include valves that are leaky or too tight and damage from high alcohol intake and thyroid disease.

Symptoms of heart failure include shortness of breath and swollen ankles. Again, these symptoms are important, and many causes of heart failure are treatable, so see your doctor.

BLOOD PRESSURE

What is high blood pressure?

One of my colleagues has spent his long career studying high blood pressure.

When I asked him the question 'what causes high blood pressure?' he could not give a simple answer. What we do know is that it isn't seen in people living a traditional lifestyle, so it is something in the secret sauce of the Western combination of dietary patterns and inactivity that is likely to be the major underlying contributor. Rarely there are other causes of hypertension, such as hormone producing tumours.

Around 34 per cent of Australians over eighteen have high blood pressure, which is a problem because untreated high blood pressure is a major cause of stroke, cardiovascular disease and dementia.

When you have your blood pressure checked, there are two numbers. The first is the systolic blood pressure, this is the peak that occurs when the ventricle in the heart contracts to push blood around the body. The second is the diastolic, when the heart is relaxed between beats. These numbers are both important. If the systolic pressure is greater than 140 mmHg or the diastolic is greater than 90 mmHg, this is considered elevated and most people will be started on treatment, although this decision will depend on the individual's actual overall cardiovascular risk.

The thing about hypertension is that unless it is extremely high, usually a systolic over 200, it doesn't cause any symptoms. Even at this level many people will still be unaware, which is why GPs routinely check blood pressure. The other important component of hypertension is that having a slightly elevated blood pressure won't cause any harm today, tomorrow or indeed for years. This doesn't mean it isn't important to treat it, because over many decades, high blood pressure can change the structure of blood vessels and increase the risk of many health conditions, including ischaemic heart disease, stroke and dementia.

For many the first line treatment is actually to look at lifestyle factors, including exercise, dietary changes and smoking cessation. Even if people are started on medications, these lifestyle factors are still important.

18

STROKE

Stroke used to be called apoplexy, which comes from the Greek for being struck down by violence. A more accurate name is a cerebrovascular accident (CVA), because a stroke occurs when there is a sudden, spontaneous injury to the brain tissue due to a blocked or ruptured blood vessel. The symptoms of stroke can include paralysis, trouble speaking and change in sensation, and will vary depending on the part of the brain that has been affected by the stroke.

Stroke is the eighth leading cause of death in Australia. Of the survivors, around 40 per cent will have a residual disability.

There are two types of stroke: ischaemic from a blocked blood vessel and haemorrhagic from a bleed. Clinically, it is very hard to tell them apart, but they are treated differently.

Ischaemic stroke

An ischaemic stroke occurs when a blood vessel in the brain is blocked. The blockage can be caused by a plaque rupture (similar to an AMI) or an embolus, a clot that has come from somewhere else. This is usually the heart or the carotid arteries, which are the large arteries in the neck that supply most of the brain or from the heart, particularly if someone has atrial fibrillation, a condition where the atria in the heart don't beat regularly which can lead to clot formation. This sudden blockage of an artery has catastrophic effects on the area downstream of the blood vessel, which is suddenly deprived of blood. As a result, this part of the brain stops working and is damaged. The aim of the immediate treatment is to try and restore blood flow as quickly as possible.

Haemorrhagic stroke

The other main type of stroke is haemorrhagic, which is when there is a bleed in the brain. This can also be age related, occurring when arteries are hardened. Less commonly, people can be born with blood vessel malformations which spontaneously burst later in life. These are called aneurisms, and can occasionally run in families. Rarely, they can be the first presentation of a brain tumour.

FAST symptoms

As with an AMI, knowing the symptoms of stroke is critical because timely treatment can have a huge impact on the level of damage caused. If you suspect you or someone else is having a stroke, you should call an ambulance to get to hospital immediately. The sooner the patient receives treatment, the better the chance of recovery.

The acronym for identifying the symptoms of stroke is FAST:

Facial drooping: Is part of their face uneven?
Arms: Are they unable to move one of their arms?
Speech: Is their speech slurred or are they using words that don't make sense?
Time: Time is critical to get treatment to save brain tissue.

Other signs include:

- weakness, numbness or paralysis of the face, arm or leg on either or both sides of the body
- difficulty speaking or understanding speech
- dizziness, loss of balance or an unexplained fall
- loss of vision, sudden blurring or decreased vision in one or both eyes
- headache, usually severe and abrupt onset or unexplained change in the pattern of headaches
- difficulty swallowing.

If you experience these symptoms or see someone with these symptoms, call an ambulance FAST.

In the emergency department

When someone is brought to the hospital emergency department with a suspected stroke, they will often go straight from the ambulance to a CT, for a scan of the brain to look for blood, or an alternate cause. On this type of scan, brain tissue is grey and blood is bright white. This is to determine whether someone has had a haemorrhagic or ischaemic stroke.

The clinicians will also be trying to establish a timeline for the onset of symptoms, trying to determine when the person was last well and exactly what time the symptoms began, as well as taking a medical history including current medications. These things are important because the treatment for ischaemic stroke is to give powerful blood thinning medications to break up the clot. These can't be used in a haemorrhagic stroke, or if the stroke happened more than four and a half hours ago (in most cases), due to the high risk of bleeding.

While this is going on, the doctors and nurses will also be making sure the patient is medically stable by checking breathing, heart rate and conscious state. In some situations, doctors will pass a narrow tube through the peripheral artery and up to the brain to retrieve the clot. If someone has had a haemorrhagic stroke, they will usually be reviewed by a neurosurgeon to determine whether they need surgery to decrease pressure in the brain.

Secondary prevention

Once the patient is stable, the next step in stroke management is to try and work out why the stroke happened so that appropriate preventative treatments can commence.

Since many strokes are caused by a build-up of atherosclerotic plaques, these investigations look at cardiovascular risk factors such as high blood pressure, diabetes and high levels of low-density lipoproteins. It is routine to start people on cholesterol-lowering medications because there is good evidence these improve survival.

A stroke can also be caused by an embolus, a clot that comes from somewhere else, which can occur when someone has atrial fibrillation, where the heartbeat is irregular and blood isn't emptied as efficiently from the heart. To look for atrial fibrillation, doctors perform 24 hours of cardiac monitoring. If atrial fibrillation is detected, blood-thinning medication will be recommended. Doctors will also perform an echocardiogram to look for structural abnormalities in the heart. There will also be an ultrasound of the carotid arteries, the major arteries in the neck to the brain, to look for a build-up of atherosclerosis as sometimes this can be removed with surgery.

19

DIABETES

Diabetes is a disease that occurs when blood glucose is too high. Based on self-reported data, around 1.2 million Australians have diabetes. However, one of the biggest problems with diabetes is that so many people don't know they have it. Most people with diabetes don't experience any symptoms until the disease is advanced. This means that for every four people with a diagnosis of diabetes, there is another person who hasn't been diagnosed.

Diabetes is diagnosed by checking the levels of glucose in the blood, usually when someone is fasting, or checking the HbA1c, which can measure the average glucose levels over three months. A normal fasting blood glucose level is less than 5.5 mmol/l. If it is between 5.5–6.9 mmol/l further testing is required, and if it is greater than 7 mmol/l, it is in the diabetic range. If someone's results are indeterminate, the next step is to do an oral glucose tolerance test. This involves fasting overnight, having a blood test then a drink with a high glucose load, followed by another blood test two hours later. This is a more sensitive way to diagnose diabetes.

There are two main types of diabetes: the first is called type 1, or juvenile diabetes, which is an autoimmune disease that usually occurs in children or young adults. In type 1 diabetes, an individual makes antibodies that act against the cells in the pancreas that make insulin. This continues until they make no insulin at all, which is rapidly fatal without insulin injections. Far more common is type 2 diabetes mellitus (T2DM), which usually occurs in adults aged 50 and older, and increases with age. Type 2 diabetes is the result of a combination of decreased insulin production and increased resistance to insulin.

How does type 2 diabetes develop?

Type 2 diabetes is caused by a combination of genetic and environmental factors. When we eat sugar or refined carbohydrates, cells in our pancreas release insulin, which tells our muscle and fat cells to absorb and use the glucose. If someone has insulin resistance, they need higher levels of insulin to manage the same glucose load. Insulin resistance is associated with increasing weight and age, and this might be mediated by inflammation from fat cells. Over time, the insulin-producing cells in the pancreas, called beta cells, wear out and can no longer produce enough insulin, so blood glucose levels begin to rise. It might be that higher levels of glucose are directly toxic to the beta cells.

What happens if we get type 2 diabetes?

Diabetes is a stealthy disease. Until blood glucose levels are very high, there are no symptoms at all, so many people can have type 2 diabetes for years and be unaware of it.

Although some people can be insulin resistant and develop diabetes despite having a low body weight, there is a direct linear relationship with diabetes and body weight. Basically, people with higher body weight have a higher chance of becoming diabetic. The pattern of fat distribution also influences the risk of diabetes, with central adiposity conferring the highest risk. As discussed in chapter 3, obesity is linked with higher levels of inflammation, and inflammation is also linked with diabetes.

The symptoms of very high blood glucose are thirst and excessive urine production, which occurs as the kidneys try to get rid of the excess glucose. These only occur when sugars are already above 15 mmol/l, so someone might have blood sugars in the diabetic range for years before they develop these symptoms. This is why people are screened for diabetes.

Diabetes shortens life expectancy because it leads to accelerated atherosclerosis, as well as kidney disease, blindness and nerve damage. It is also an important risk factor for dementia, as it can cause damage to small and large blood vessels in the brain. It usually takes around 10–15 years of diabetes for these complications to develop, but sadly I have met too many people who only learn they have diabetes because they already have a secondary complication.

MANAGING TYPE 2 DIABETES

One of the challenges in management of type 2 diabetes is that when someone has had this condition for a long time, particularly if they have secondary complications, it is actually possible to do real harm with aggressive blood sugar control. The UKPDS study recruited people with newly diagnosed diabetes and randomised them to either aggressive blood sugar control, aiming for a measure of less than 6 mmol/l, or a blood sugar level of less than 15mmol/l, which was standard control at the time. After ten years, the intensive control group had a reduction in microvascular complications related to diabetes. This study was published in 1998 and had a huge influence on practice, with more aggressive treatment of diabetes becoming routine.

In 2008, another study was published that led to another major shift in management. The ACCORD trial recruited 10,250 participants who had long-standing type 2 diabetes (for an average of ten years), and they were randomised to aggressive blood sugar control or usual management. This trial was stopped after 3.7 years, instead of the planned five, because of increased deaths due to cardiovascular disease.

The ACCORD trial has made those of us who manage people with long-standing diabetes change our practice, particularly to avoid the risk of hypoglycaemia, or low blood sugar from medication. With patients who are older adults, particularly if they are frail, I aim for symptomatic blood sugar control with levels between 7–15 mmol/l, because current evidence indicates this is safer. Part of the reason for this is that people with long-standing diabetes, particularly if it has been poorly controlled, are often at high risk of hypoglycaemic unawareness, meaning that blood sugars can get dangerously low before they are aware there is a problem. Diabetes management needs to be tailored to each individual patient, and it is best to discuss this with your doctor.

Diabetes treatment

Sometimes a person only learns of their diabetes due to a secondary complication, like a heart attack. If diabetes is mild, the first step is to look at diet and exercise. There is still some controversy about the optimal diet for type 2 diabetes, particularly around low-carbohydrate diets, but the dietary principles outlined in chapter 8 and exercise in chapter 9 are a reasonable start.

If blood sugar levels are not controlled with diet and exercise, the next step is tablet medication. The first medication prescribed is usually metformin. Metformin decreases glucose production by the liver and increases glucose uptake by the muscles. It also has a positive effect on lipid profiles. Metformin is generally very safe and well-tolerated, with no risk of low blood sugar, and can cause weight loss. There are many other second line tablets that can be used if Metformin alone is insufficient to control diabetes. If tablets are insufficient, people usually start on insulin injections.

I have seen a handful of patients who have reversed their type 2 diabetes with diet, but it has been rare. In a study of over 5000 people with type 2 diabetes, half were randomised for either an intensive lifestyle intervention program or standard diabetes education. The intensive program involved a strict calorie target of 1200–1500 calories per day for those who weighed less than 114 kilograms and 1500–1800 for those who weighed greater than 114 kilograms. They were also given a target of 175 minutes of exercise a week equivalent to brisk walking.

After one year, 11.5 per cent of people in the intensive group had achieved partial or complete remission of their diabetes, compared to 2 per cent of the standard education group, although at four years, that 11.5 per cent had fallen to 7 per cent. This was higher in people who managed to maintain weight loss. Both time-restricted eating and a 4:3 regime for intermittent fasting have shown improved insulin sensitivity, although in a study comparing caloric restriction and intermittent fasting, there was no difference in outcomes between the two groups, with both losing weight.

While we do have evidence that it is possible to reverse type 2 diabetes with diet, I think that the take home from these studies is that change needs to be sustainable. Very few people are able to seriously restrict calories for a long period of time – it's hard and unpleasant. For some people fasting will be easier, but that doesn't work for everyone either. Making significant lifestyle changes can have huge health benefits, but they need to fit in with your own life so they are sustainable.

THE METABOLIC SYNDROME

We are all encouraged to have regular check-ups to measure blood pressure, cholesterol and blood sugar, especially after the age of 50, and for good reason. Many of the diseases of ageing are related to what is called the metabolic syndrome, which is the presence of multiple, related risk factors including abnormal blood lipid profiles, high blood pressure, abdominal obesity and impaired glucose tolerance.

As these factors most frequently occur together, it is very hard to work out causal relationships. For example, do people gain weight because they have insulin resistance, or do they develop insulin resistance because they have gained weight?

Metabolic syndrome is present in around 40 per cent of people aged over 60 in the USA, and figures in the UK and Australia are likely to be similar.

Having metabolic syndrome isn't a disease per se, but it can lead to developing multiple diseases, including heart disease, stroke, dementia, diabetes, kidney disease and many, many others. Unsurprisingly, it is also associated with inflammation.

Often medications are needed to manage these conditions, but making lifestyle changes can be critical to modifying our risk of metabolic syndromes and the diseases it is likely to cause.

20

CANCER

Cancer is not one single disease, it is caused by genetic mutations that lead to a loss of checks and balances on cell division.

As we saw in part 1, the adult human body has around 37 trillion cells, all originating from that first fertilised ova dividing over and over again. Every time a cell divides, there are errors in DNA replication. Many of these will have no effect at all, but an error in a gene that controls DNA repair (or replication itself) can start the cascade of errors that becomes a cancer. Cancer is more common with age simply because our cells have divided more times so there is more opportunity for error.

Some cancer cells aren't all that different to the ones they arose from; these ones are often stuck where they first grew, and may never actually cause any trouble at all. Some cancer cells rapidly accumulate mutations that enable them to spread throughout the body, causing disease in distant organs and eventually death. Cancer, however, can behave very differently in different people, which is one reason researching treatment is so difficult.

Screening for cancer

Cancer incidence increases with age, as our cells have divided more times. We are able to screen for some cancers, such as breast and cervical cancer. Screening means looking for a disease when there are no symptoms. There are three screening programs that are recommended at the population level in Australia: bowel, breast and cervical. These cancer screening programs are recommended because they have been widely studied and shown to be effective. Some screening programs have been extremely successful. The widespread rollout of pap smears to look for cancerous or precancerous cells on the cervix has dramatically reduced deaths from cervical cancer, as it can be identified and treated early. This screening is recommended for women aged 25–74. Even though there is now a vaccine for human papilloma virus, which causes most of these cancers, and it is likely to almost disappear, screening is still recommended.

In Australia, invitations for breast screening are sent to women aged 50–74, although women aged 40–50 are also eligible, as are women over 74 who choose to undertake screening. Since breast screening was introduced in 1991, there has been a marked decrease in mortality from breast cancer, although this is also the result of better treatment.

One of the challenges in screening programs is that our imaging techniques are not perfect, even for breast cancer screening. When women have a mammogram, 11 per cent will be recalled for additional investigations, but only around 1 per cent of women screened will actually have breast cancer, meaning that most of those recalled for further investigations don't have cancer. This false positive can cause significant stress. Screening can also miss a cancer. If you have had a mammogram that was normal, but you notice a new lump or other change in your breast, you should still see your doctor.

When you turn 50 you get a special birthday gift from the government: a kit so you can send away a sample of your poo to check for blood. This is because colorectal cancer causes the second highest number of deaths after lung cancer, and around 90 per cent of these deaths are preventable with early detection. If this test is positive, the next step is a colonoscopy to look for any cancerous lesions inside the bowel. Again, if there actually are concerning symptoms, such as weight loss or bleeding from the anus, these still need to be discussed with your doctor.

Other types of cancer screening are still controversial. Screening for prostate cancer has shown only a modest benefit for context, prostate cancer is extremely common in men as they get older, and for most it will remained confined to the prostate and never cause any problems,

Other than for breast, bowel and cervical cancer, there are no other coordinated national screening programs for the general population. Although many people do undergo skin checks, there is insufficient evidence that this impacts the rate of mortality from melanoma. Some people, if they are at a particularly high risk, such as those with a strong family history, may benefit from additional screening for certain cancers; they should discuss this with their doctor.

SYMPTOMS YOU SHOULD NEVER IGNORE

- Unexplained weight loss
- Persistent night sweats and fever
- A new breast or underarm lump or a change in the skin, particularly if the skin looks dimpled like an orange
- Any post-menopausal vaginal bleeding, or pre-menopausal bleeding between periods, including bleeding after sex

- Bleeding from the anus, whether it is in, on or after the faeces
- A change in bowel habits (for example, if you've always been regular and become constipated)
- A new mole or a mole that is growing and changing shape or colour

If something feels off and is bothering or worrying you, it is worth checking in with your doctor. You are the world expert on your body. We all worry about feeling foolish because there is nothing wrong, but that is a far better feeling than lying awake in bed at night worrying you have a disease.

Cancer treatment

Cancer is one word for a disease that occurs in almost every part of the body. It can also behave very differently, making it very hard to give a succinct summary of the treatment. If a tumour is early stage, and it isn't around critical structures, surgery is an option, and in the best case this is curable. Radiotherapy utilises radiation to target the cancer cells, which are more sensitive to the damage this causes. Chemotherapy uses many different drugs that are toxic to cells in order to kill the cancer cells. As with radiotherapy, cancer cells are more sensitive to this than regular cells because they are less able to repair the damage. For some types of blood cancer, like leukaemia, chemotherapy alone is used.

There have also been some novel developments in cancer treatment involving drugs that target immune markers on tumour cells. This is a promising new area of cancer treatment.

Cancer treatment is complex and there is no one-size-fits-all. The gold standard of cancer treatment is a multidisciplinary approach, with good communication between surgeons, oncologists and radiation oncologists so that the optimal treatment can be agreed on.

If you are unlucky enough to have cancer or to have a loved one with cancer, it is very important to feel like you are able to ask your treating team lots of questions. It is incredibly hard to take in information when you are dealing with a terrible emotional shock like a cancer diagnosis. Although doctors are taught communication skills, we are so used to speaking to other health professionals that we sometimes forget that the words we are using are medical jargon and not common knowledge. If you don't understand something your doctor says, it isn't you, it is your doctor not explaining it well enough. It is okay to keep asking for clarification.

21

MUSCULOSKELETAL DISORDERS

Our bone and muscle health are essential to enjoying a long life.

Not all conditions that are common in older age will directly kill you, but this doesn't mean they aren't significant. It is also incredibly important to understand and manage conditions that have an adverse effect on physical functioning. These include arthritis, osteoporosis and sarcopenia (loss of muscle strength and function).

Arthritis

Arthritis is a general term that refers to joint damage. It falls into two categories: osteoarthritis and inflammatory arthritis. According to Arthritis Australia, there are four million Australians living with arthritis, and these numbers will rise as the average population age increases.

Osteoarthritis

Osteoarthritis (OA) is associated with the 'wear and tear' that we see in older age. OA varies hugely from person to person: some people will show significant damage on X-ray, others will have significant pain but there will be little to see on X-ray. OA can affect almost any joint, although the more common ones are the base of the thumb, the fingers, the hips and the knees. Severe OA can limit activities of daily living and is a cause of significant disability for older adults. Women are more likely than men to get OA, and this becomes more likely with older age, obesity and smoking. Interestingly, the repetitive stress of running is not associated with OA, which may be due to runners having good muscle strength.

Treatments for osteoarthritis

One of the treatments for OA is joint replacement, but even with severe OA there is evidence that physical therapies can make a huge difference. There is strong evidence that land-based exercise can lead to decreased pain for people with OA, even if the disease is so advanced that they are waiting for a knee replacement.

There is also evidence that, for those who are overweight, weight loss can help reduce symptoms and slow disease progression.

Inflammatory arthritis

Inflammatory arthritis is usually caused by joint damage due to an overactive immune system. There are many types, and the treatments can vary significantly depending on the cause, which is why it is important to get a proper assessment with your doctor.

Rheumatoid arthritis

Rheumatoid arthritis occurs when the immune system loses regulation and actually starts to attack the joints, leading to swelling, redness, pain and stiffness. Over a long period of time, this causes damage to the joints. We now have disease modifying treatments that can usually control the symptoms and prevent long-term damage.

Other autoimmune-based arthritis

Other autoimmune diseases that cause arthritis include lupus, ankylosing spondylitis and seronegative arthritis (so-named because, clinically, it is similar to rheumatoid arthritis but has different blood markers).

Gout

Gout and pseudogout also fall into the category of inflammatory arthritis, but they are not autoimmune diseases. They occur when there is a build-up of crystals in the joints, which then leads to immune system activation, which results in swelling, redness and intense pain. Some people have a particularly strong genetic predisposition to gout due to genetic differences in protein metabolism. This can be treated with medication.

CHRONIC PAIN

Two of my brothers have chronic back pain. Tom has a condition called ankylosing spondylitis. This is an autoimmune disease where the immune system causes inflammation, and eventually damage to the sacroiliac joints between the pelvis and the spine. Left unchecked, this can cause severe damage. My other brother, James, has the far more common 'musculoskeletal back pain'; there isn't a clear physical lesion that corresponds to the pain he experiences.

For Tom, the brother with 'ank spond', the autoimmune disease, treatment is easy. He has a monthly injection of an immune-modulating drug that controls his symptoms. James, the brother with the more common type of back pain, saw many physiotherapists, doctors and osteopaths before finding a workable solution for his back pain, which involves a regular exercise routine. James knows that if he stops doing this, his back pain can flare. It has taken him years to reach a point where his pain is manageable, but he has stayed active through this time.

In my work in pain, I am incredibly lucky to work with an interdisciplinary team with a physiotherapist, psychologist, occupational therapist, anaesthetists and a social worker. This is because for most people with chronic pain, it isn't as simple as finding a 'spot' and fixing it. Chronic pain is often the result of central sensitisation, where the pain pathways in the brain become overactive and start to sense normal stimuli as painful. There is also often a component of fear, where people being scared to try a movement that causes pain means they are causing damage. For most people with chronic pain, treatment will involve physiotherapy to help strengthen muscles and to learn to move without fear, and a psychologist for cognitive behavioural therapy (CBT). Because chronic pain is usually due to abnormal processing of pain signals in the brain, CBT helps people relearn ways to manage this. This is the most evidence-based treatment for chronic pain. While chronic pain can be incredibly disabling and difficult to manage, there are treatments available and it is worth speaking to your general practitioner about referral to an interdisciplinary clinic to get the right treatment. There is usually no easy fix for chronic pain, but doing the work can lead to a huge improvement in quality of life.

Osteosarcopenia

The most common reason older adults are admitted to trauma units in hospital isn't car crashes. It's falling from standing height, which is the cause of 62.5 per cent of trauma admissions for people over 65. We all have stumbles, but frail older adults are far less able to recover from these before they fall completely, and when they do hit the ground, they are more likely to sustain a serious injury. Older adults are more likely to get fractures because of weakened bone (osteoporosis) and loss of muscle (sarcopenia) – conditions that so commonly occur together that clinicians are referring to them as osteosarcopenia.

Osteoporosis – our bones are alive

Osteoporosis literally means porous bone, and occurs when the bone becomes brittle and vulnerable to fracture.

Osteoporosis can be identified using a bone density scan, which is a special kind of X-ray. It can also be diagnosed on the basis of a fragility fracture, which is a break or crack from a relatively small force, such as a fall from a standing position or a vertebrae collapsing under its own weight, for example.

It is difficult to estimate the proportion of the population with osteoporosis because there are no symptoms other than a minimal trauma fracture, and many people don't have screening. However, it is estimated that around two in five women and one in four men will experience a fracture in their lifetime, although not all of these will be due to osteoporosis.

Although the risk of fracture increases as bone density decreases, most fragility fractures actually occur in people with osteopenia. Osteopenia means that bone density is less than average, but not thin enough to classify as osteoporosis. There are more people in this group and so more fractures. This also highlights that the mineral density of bone isn't the whole story: as a living tissue, bone strength is influenced by many of the factors that affect body health as a whole.

Sarcopenia – it's not just about the bones

Bone is an active, living tissue that is highly responsive to the muscles and other connective tissue around it. This is why using our muscles can actually stimulate bone to get stronger, and why losing muscle contributes to loss of bone strength.

Sarcopenia is the name given to the loss of muscle volume, strength and power that occurs with age and can be measured with the same type of X-ray that measures bone density. Weaker muscles obviously increase the risk of falls, and there is a higher possibility that these falls will result in a fracture. If sarcopenia is severe, it can actually result in a loss of function, leading to dependence.

The most important risk factor for sarcopenia is inactivity. Women are also at increased risk of both osteoporosis and sarcopenia because in our twenties and thirties, when bone and muscle peak, our peak is lower than men. We do lose bone and muscle with age, but optimising lifestyle factors can delay this.

Bone and muscle need to be treated together

The traditional approach to treating osteoporosis has been calcium and vitamin D supplementation, plus medication to decrease bone resorption. While calcium and vitamin D play an important role in bone health, the value of taking supplements for protection is contentious, particularly because calcium may increase the risk of cardiac events, although this is far from certain. Prospective trials using calcium and vitamin D for fracture prevention have had mixed results, and their role in fracture prevention is still highly debated. One caveat on this is that if people have measurably low levels of vitamin D, it should still be treated; this blood test will usually be ordered by your doctor.

Bone health is not just as simple as taking a tablet. Weight training and exercise with impact are also important (see chapter 9). Although bone density can definitely respond to weight training, it's not clear whether osteoporosis can be completely prevented. Staying active to prevent sarcopenia is one of the most powerful tools we have to maintain our health well into older age.

22

PREVENTION

All for one and one for all!

In the previous chapters I have looked at the main diseases that become more common with age, briefly describing symptoms, diagnosis and treatment. But one thing I haven't done is list risk factors for the individual conditions.

Risk factors are physiological characteristics or behaviours that increase a person's risk of developing a disease. One of the problems in the current model of preventative health is that prevention is often single disease focused, and single risk factor focused. Sometimes we can draw a straight line between a disease and its cause. For example, the lifetime risk of lung cancer for smokers is 20–40 times higher than for non-smokers. Despite this, not all smokers will get lung cancer or chronic obstructive pulmonary disease (COPD), and we don't know why. And some non-smokers will get lung cancer and COPD, and we don't know why either.

Our health care system and research framework developed over the last few hundred years. When the hospital where I work was founded, the most common cause of death was infectious diseases.

The only 'treatment' for a heart attack was bed rest. Now we have specialised treatments for different conditions that are delivered by specialists in that area. If I experience a sudden blockage of a coronary artery, I will be grateful to have a skilled cardiologist who has extensive specialist training to unblock it. The problem is that all of the chronic conditions in this book are associated with the same underlying processes. When research is conducted that only lists one outcome, such as heart disease or stroke or diabetes, this ignores the fact that these conditions are all associated and share many common pathways.

Prevention doesn't mean choosing the disease that you are most concerned about and deciding to avoid it. The beauty of making lifestyle changes is that since there is so much commonality in the underlying processes, particularly inflammation, making a positive lifestyle change will improve the chances of a long and healthy life by reducing the risk of chronic disease overall.

We know that certain risk factors will dramatically increase the odds of getting certain age-related diseases, such as heart disease, sarcopenia, diabetes, osteoarthritis and dementia, but the good news is that almost all of these conditions are related to the same underlying processes, and risk can be modified with lifestyle changes.

For example, peripheral vascular disease (where arteries in the leg become blocked), ischaemic heart disease and stroke all share the same risk factors:

- high blood pressure
- poor blood lipid profiles (including high cholesterol)
- smoking
- diabetes

Each of these risk factors, in turn, is affected by our lifestyle (our diet, activity levels, stress levels and the quality of our sleep). And the great news is that improving any of these can reduce our risk of disease.

The value of a family doctor

One of the reasons everyone needs a good GP or family doctor is that they have an overview of your lifestyle choices and your health over time. Regular check-ups with your GP to assess your risk factors and offer lifestyle advice and medications are the thing that may prevent heart disease in the first place. As the Royal Australian College of General Practitioners says, 'A GP is your specialist in life.'

CONCLUSION

I don't know how long my life will be and neither do you.
I do know that today I will eat food that is nourishing, go
to bed early to get a good night's sleep, move fast enough
to feel alive, look around me and see the beauty in my
world and cherish those I love.

If there is one take-home message from this book it is this: you don't have to choose between things that make you feel better now and longevity. Choosing to feel engaged, motivated, strong and rested now is a pathway to living as long and as well as possible. Life is too short for choices that are unpleasant and restrictive, it is too short to spend time waiting for something to happen before you start enjoying yourself. Life is what is happening now.

This doesn't mean that we forget about the future. I hope that this book has also sparked you to think about what truly matters to you and what drives you. Just as our mind allows us to revisit the past, it also allows us to imagine the future.

So what do you want for your future? While there are no guarantees that things will work out exactly as planned – in fact, they almost certainly won't – thinking about what matters to you and what you would like your life to be when you are in your eighties, nineties and beyond will affect the decisions you make today. These might be decisions about where you live, how much money you want to save before retirement or which friendships you most value.

It's all about inflammation

Think back to the last time you had the flu – remember the lethargy, the aches, the weakness and foggy head? This is how you feel when your body has high levels of inflammation. Of all the biomarkers related to health, inflammation is the one that is most consistent. Of course, a robust immune system is essential to fight off infection, but it is decades of slightly higher than average immune activation that has been strongly linked to poorer health. Our immune function is also influenced by almost everything we do, from going to bed at a reasonable time at night, to the food we eat, to finding a fulfilling and meaningful role in life.

From a biological point of view, wellbeing depends on our body's ability to minimise baseline levels of inflammation. We also want to encourage our cells into repair pathways, to optimise their chance to recover from everyday metabolic stress.

Just as health has physical, mental, cognitive and emotional aspects, all of these will ultimately affect the same underlying biological pathways. One question I can't answer is whether one aspect is more important than another. All of these factors are interdependent, and can influence each other in positive or negative ways. To take just one example, optimists are more likely to take their blood pressure medications and to exercise, which contributes to lower levels of inflammation. Changing diet to include vegetables and whole foods to improve mood could decrease the risk of dementia and increase the likelihood of living longer. Making social connection with people who give you emotional nourishment could have a positive effect on your cortisol levels, thus decreasing the risk of cardiovascular disease.

One of the most confronting truths about prevention is that it might not work. Life and health are not always fair. Cultivating optimism, eating delicious and nutritious foods and spending time with people you love are rewards in themselves. Prevention is an attractive concept, but we need to focus on the here and now. We also need to confront our own mortality. The choices you make can have a huge influence on your future health. But they can also have a huge influence on how much you enjoy today.

SAMPLE RECIPES

When I create a recipe, my primary goal is to make something that I will enjoy eating. Of course there are other considerations. Nutrition is one of my key strategies for enjoying life, so I follow the food principles outlined in chapter 8 – all whole ingredients, with lots of plants and a little meat or fish. Most of the time I am preparing dinner in a hurry for my family, so many of these recipes can be made quickly, but I also love having a little more time on weekends to create something special.

If you like these recipes, there are more as part of my online course at www.projectthreesixtwelve.com.

Main meals

Roast chicken with Puy lentils

This is such a delicious way to cook chicken and lentils, it always seems to stay really moist, and cooking the chicken over the lentils means that the lentils take on the flavour of the chicken as well. I really love Puy lentils, they maintain their shape really well, which gives them a great texture and they also have a peppery after taste.

Serves: 4–5
Prep time: 15 minutes
Cooking time: 1 hour 10 minutes, plus resting time

1 leek, white and light green parts only, finely sliced and washed
4 tomatoes, diced
1 cup Puy lentils
2 garlic heads, peeled, or 20 garlic cloves
1 bunch of thyme
1 whole chicken (2 kg, preferably free range)
1 cup frozen peas
lemon
extra virgin olive oil
½ cup verjuice

Preheat the oven to 220°C (200°C fan-forced).

Scatter the leek and tomatoes in the bottom of a large roasting dish. Place the lentils into the dish, add 2 ½ cups water and stir through. Scatter over the garlic cloves and place 4–5 thyme sprigs in the dish.

Stuff the chicken with the lemon and remaining thyme sprigs.

Rub the chicken with olive oil and season with sea salt and freshly ground black pepper.

Place a roasting rack on top of the roasting dish. Place the chicken, breast-side up, on the roasting rack and place foil over the chicken. Roast for 30 minutes then remove the baking tray from the oven. Take the foil off and pour the verjuice over the chicken.

Reduce the heat to 200°C (180°C fan-forced) and place the baking tray back in the oven, uncovered, for 30 minutes. Remove from oven and place chicken, breast-side down, on a board to cool for 30 minutes.

Stir the peas into the lentil mixture then place back in the oven for 10 minutes, then serve.

NOTE: If there are leftover lentils, they are even more delicious the next day!

Corn fritters with avocado salsa

This is a fast weeknight dinner staple at our house. I usually have it with some poached eggs and leafy greens.

Makes: 8
Prep time: 10 minutes
Cooking time: 10 minutes

70 ml milk (cow's milk or soy)
2 eggs
3 tablespoons extra virgin olive oil
125 g wholemeal or plain flour
1 teaspoon smoked paprika
1 teaspoon baking soda
pinch of sea salt
2 spring onions, finely sliced
1 × 420 g tinned corn
haloumi, grilled (optional)

AVOCADO SALSA
1 avocado
juice of 1 lime
1 tomato, finely chopped

Whisk the milk, eggs and olive oil in a bowl and set aside. Combine the flour, paprika, baking soda and sea salt in a separate bowl. Add the wet ingredients to the dry ingredients and mix until combined. Add in corn and spring onion and mix well.

Heat a frying pan with a tablespoon of olive oil and heat over medium heat.

Take a serving spoon of the mixture and add to the pan. Cook for 3 minutes each side or until golden and cooked through. Remove and keep warm.

For the avocado salsa, mash the avocado then add the lime juice and tomato and mix until combined.

Divide the fritters among plates and top with the avocado salsa to serve. You can also add some grilled haloumi, if you like.

Coconut curry fish pie

This is one of my favourites for the winter months – the warm, aromatic flavours are perfect for a cold day.

Makes: 6–8 serves
Prep time: 20 minutes
Cooking time: 45 minutes

400 g desiree potato, peeled

1 teaspoon fenugreek

20 g piece of ginger, finely chopped

15 g piece of turmeric, finely chopped

2 lemongrass stalks, white part only, roughly chopped and crushed with a pestle or the side of a large knife

1 long red chilli, deseeded and chopped

30 g oil

20 g water

400 g salmon, cut into 2 × 2 cm pieces

200 g white fish, cut into 2 × 2 pieces

200 g green prawns, peeled, deveined and heads removed

280 ml coconut milk

1 tablespoon coconut sugar

1 tablespoon fish sauce

2 tomatoes, finely chopped

2 handfuls of spinach leaves

canola oil, for cooking

Steam the potatoes until soft.

Meanwhile, add canola oil to a non-stick frying pan and place over low heat. Gently toast fenugreek for a few minutes or until aromatic. Remove from the pan and place in a mortar and pestle.

To make the curry paste, place the ginger, turmeric, lemongrass, chilli, oil and water with the fenugreek in the mortar and pestle and grind to a fine paste. Alternatively blend in a food processor.

Heat some canola oil in a large non-stick saucepan over medium–high heat. Add the curry paste to the saucepan and cook for 1–2 minutes then take the saucepan off the heat.

Preheat the oven to 200°C (180°C fan-forced).

Coat the fish and prawns in the curry paste and place in a baking dish. Place coconut milk, coconut sugar and fish sauce in a bowl and whisk until combined. Add the mixture, tomato and spinach to the baking dish. Mash the potatoes then cover the fish mixture completely. Bake for 45 minutes.

Homemade chicken stock

My children refuse to eat anything but homemade chicken stock. It really is completely different to the ones on the supermarket shelves, far more flavoursome and less salty. While there are some better quality ones available, they are not as cheap as making it yourself. I use my slow cooker for this, but it is also possible to do this on the stove. I also keep roast chicken remains frozen to save space, alternately you can ask your butcher for some bones. Any vegetables can be put it, especially if they are looking a bit sad!

Makes: 1.5 L
Prep time: 10 minutes
Cooking time: 2–4 hours

½ chicken carcass, broken up
½ onion, coarsely chopped
1 carrot, coarsely chopped
1 celery stick, coarsely chopped
fresh or dried herbs (I prefer thyme and rosemary, but use whatever I have
    available)
½ teaspoon sea salt

Place all ingredients in a slow cooker and cover with around 1.5 L water. Slow cook on high for 4 hours. Alternatively, place all ingredients in a saucepan over high heat. Bring to the boil, then turn the heat to low and simmer for 1 ½–2 hours.

Strain the stock into a large saucepan and use at once or store in an airtight container in the fridge for 4–5 days or freeze for up to 6 months.

Minestrone

This is just absolutely jam-packed with vegetables. I usually make it with my homemade chicken stock, but you can substitute Massel stock cubes.

Makes: 1.5 L
Prep time: 20 minutes + soaking overnight
Cooking time: 45 minutes

1 cup dried cannellini beans
2 × 400 g tinned diced tomatoes (no added salt)
2 carrots, finely diced
2 zucchinis, finely diced
2 celery sticks, finely diced
1 onion, finely diced
2 garlic cloves, crushed
homemade chicken stock (see page 286)
handful of shredded cabbage
handful of shredded baby spinach leaves
1 bunch of basil leaves

Place the cannellini beans in a large bowl, cover with water and soak overnight.

Heat olive oil in a large saucepan over medium heat. Add the onion and garlic and cook until onion softens. Add the carrots, zucchini and celery and more olive oil, if necessary, and cook for 7 minutes or until vegetables are slightly tender.

Add the tomatoes, cannellini beans and chicken stock, bring to the boil, then turn the heat to low and simmer for 45 minutes.

Turn off the heat then add the cabbage, spinach and basil leaves.

Divide the soup among bowls and serve with chunks of toasted sourdough.

NOTE: I like to top the sourdough with chilli and parmesan and toast it in the oven on 200°C (180°C fan-forced) for 15–20 minutes.

Salads and veggies

Herby potato salad

Potatoes have had a bad reputation, because they are high in carbo-hydrates. While it is true that we are able to break down starch very fast, when we cook and cool potatoes, the starch is trans-formed into resistant starch, which acts like fibre and becomes a valuable fuel source for our microbiome.

Serves: 5–6 as a side
Prep time: 15 minutes
Cooking time: 15 minutes

1 kg small white potatoes, skin on
30 ml verjuice
30 ml extra virgin olive oil
1 bunch of mint leaves, finely chopped
1 bunch flat-leaf parsley, finely chopped
1 × 110 g jar capers in vinegar, drained
2 anchovy fillets

Place the potatoes in a saucepan of water, bring to the boil, then turn the heat to low and simmer for around 15 minutes or until tender.

Meanwhile, to make the dressing, add the verjuice and olive oil in a small bowl and mix until combined. Add the anchovies and use a spoon to break them up.

Drain the potatoes then while the potatoes are still warm, mix through the dressing. After 20 minutes or when the potatoes have cooled, add in herbs and capers, mix well and serve.

Honey- and Dijon mustard-glazed Brussels sprouts

Brussels sprouts have a bad reputation, and they certainly aren't nice when they are steamed or boiled until they are soggy. The key to preparing Brussels sprouts so they are delicious is to make sure they have a slightly crispy texture. With the addition of honey and Dijon, I challenge anyone to still claim they don't like Brussels sprouts.

Serves: 4–5 as a side
Prep time: 5 minutes
Cooking time: 25 minutes

300 g Brussels sprouts, trimmed
1 teaspoon Dijon mustard
juice of ½ lemon
1 teaspoon honey
2 tablespoons extra virgin olive oil

Preheat the oven to 200°C (180°C fan-forced). Line a baking tray with baking paper.

Place olive oil, honey and Dijon mustard in a large bowl and mix until well combined. Add the Brussels sprouts and toss to coat.

Place the Brussels sprouts on the prepared tray and bake for 25 minutes or until slightly browned.

Pear, rocket and parmesan salad

Rocket has such a strong peppery taste and the sweetness of the pear is an excellent balance, which is why this combination is a classic.

Serves: 2–4 as a side
Prep time: 5 minutes

¼ cup extra virgin olive oil
juice of ½ lemon
1 tablespoon honey
2 Packham pears, cored and thinly sliced
150 g rocket leaves
¼ cup shaved parmesan
¼ cup crushed walnuts

To make the dressing, place olive oil, lemon juice and honey in a small bowl and mix until combined.

In a serving bowl, add pear, rocket and dressing and mix to combine.

Top the salad with the parmesan and walnuts.

Lunch and snacks

Oat and chia porridge

This is my morning go-to, high in fibre and good fat to keep me full.

Serves: 1
Prep time: 5 minutes
Cooking time: 2 ½ minutes

2 tablespoons chia seeds
⅓ cup oats
½ pear, cored and diced
1 tablespoon tahini
1 teaspoon raw cacao powder
pine nuts, to serve

Place the chia seeds in a bowl, cover with ½ cup water and soak for five minutes.

Cover and microwave on high for 90 seconds. Stir then micro-wave for an additional 60 seconds.

Add in the tahini and cacao powder and mix until well combined. Scatter over the pine nuts and serve.

Banana bread

Let's be honest, most banana bread is actually cake. This recipe is actually healthy since it's just sweetened with bananas, and one of my most requested by friends.

Serves: 7–8
Prep time: 10 minutes
Cooking time: 30–40 minutes

20 g chia seeds
50 g water
220 g wholemeal flour
70 g oats
1 teaspoon ground cinnamon
10 g bicarbonate soda
2 very ripe bananas
2 eggs
100 ml olive oil
30 g honey

Preheat the oven to 180°C (160°C fan-forced) and grease a small loaf tin.

Place the chia seeds in a bowl, cover with the water and soak for 5 minutes.

Place the flour, oats, cinnamon and bicarbonate soda in a large bowl and mix to combine.

Mash the bananas then place in a separate bowl with the eggs, olive oil and honey and mix until well combined. Add the chia seeds and water and mix to combine.

Mix the dry and wet ingredients together then place in the prepared loaf tin.

Bake for 40 minutes or until a skewer inserted in the centre of the loaf comes out clean.

NOTE: You can also replace the oats with crushed walnuts, if you like.

Sauerkraut on toast

This is my favourite quick, go-to lunch. I actually make my own sauerkraut, it is as easy as grating the cabbage, massaging it with salt then letting it sit in a fermentation crock for a couple of weeks. It is much cheaper than buying it ready-made.

Serves: 1
Prep time: 5 minutes

2 slices sourdough bread, toasted
½ avocado, mashed
1 handful of sauerkraut
pepitas

Drizzle some olive oil on the toasted bread. Top with avocado and sauerkraut then scatter over the pepitas and serve immediately.

Baked quince

I love quince, it is just magical how the colour changes from white to a deep pink when cooked. These quinces make an excellent addition to porridge or a decadent after-dinner treat.

Serves: 5
Prep time: 15 minutes
Cooking time: 3 hours

3 quinces, skin on, quartered and pips removed
1 tablespoon honey
1 tablespoon caster sugar
1 cinnamon stick
1 bay leaf
pinch of freshly ground black pepper
zest and juice of 1 lemon
Greek-style yoghurt or coconut yoghurt, to serve (optional)
vanilla bean paste, to serve (optional)

Preheat the oven to 170°C (150°C fan-forced).

Wash the quince and rub with a rough cloth to remove fuzz. Cut the quince quarters in half again. Place them in a baking dish that has a lid. Drizzle with the honey and sprinkle with the caster sugar.

Add the cinnamon stick, bay leaf, pepper, lemon zest and juice and ½ cup water and mix the ingredients.

Cover the baking dish with the lid and bake for 3 hours or until quinces are soft if you stick a fork in.

Serve with a dollop of yoghurt and a drizzle of vanilla bean paste, if desired.

ACKNOWLEDGEMENTS

Writing a book was never really a dream of mine, because it seemed too much to hope for. To me, understanding science makes the world a little more magical, and I am still pinching myself that I have the opportunity to share this with the world.

I would like to thank the team at Pan Macmillan, especially Ingrid Ohlsson, Alex Lloyd and Miriam Cannell. A special thank you to Katie Crawford, who I asked for advice about writing a book and instantly offered to take a look at my outline, which prompted me to learn what an outline was and write one!

My wonderful agent Margaret Gee has been a fantastic support and an early champion of this book.

Professor Felice Jacka and Dr Sarah McKay provided invaluable advice about the process of writing a book.

The best parts of researching this book was interviewing so many wonderful scientists about their work. All of these people were so incredibly generous with their time, and the book would not be nearly so rich or accurate without them, including Professor Linda Fried, Professor Cynthia Kenyon and Professor Judith Campisi. I am also grateful to the people, mostly anonymous, who shared their own health and life stories with me, including my patients who are so generous with sharing their wisdom.

I would like to thank my PhD supervisors, Professor Kwang Lim and Professor Ruth Hubbard, for introducing me to new concepts around health and ageing, helping with career opportunities and being very understanding when I was a little slow completing my thesis because I decided to write a book in the middle of it! I also want to thank Professor Michael Murray who was the reason I decided to specialise in geriatric medicine.

I still can't quite believe I decided to write a book when I was working as a doctor, halfway through a PhD and had three small children, the youngest only eight months old. I need to thank my children, Lily, Harvey and Arthur, for being so understanding for all the time Mummy had to disappear to write. I could not have done this without my village, and I need to acknowledge my mother and my mother-in-law who help with childcare. My children have also thrived with the wonderful babysitters and educators who are also part of the village which has enabled me to write this book while knowing that my children are loved.

I have saved the most important thank you for last: my husband, Michael. From the time I wrote my first ever article in 2016, he has been an absolute, unwavering support. He has gone above and beyond to support my writing, from editing my clumsy initial articles, to creating a personal website for me and a website to go with this book. Without his practical and emotional support, I could never have done this.

ENDNOTES

Chapter 1: Life expectancy

5. Fast-forward 160 years and infant mortality . . . : *Levels and Trends in Child Mortality*. United Nation Children's Fund. 2019.

Chapter 2: Cellular ageing

12. The incidence of CHIP increases with . . . : Jaiswal S, Natarajan P, Silver AJ, et al. 'Clonal Hematopoiesis and Risk of Atherosclerotic Cardiovascular Disease'. *New England Journal of Medicine*. 2017;377(2):111-121.

14. In studies of centenarians, greater telomere . . . : Blackburn EH, Epel ES, Lin J. 'Human telomere biology: A contributory and interactive factor in aging, disease risks, and protection'. *Science*. 2015;350(6265):1193-1198.

15. The pattern of DNA methylation changes . . . : Horvath S, Raj K. 'DNA methylation-based biomarkers and the epigenetic clock theory of ageing'. *Nature Reviews Genetics*. 2018;19(6):371-384.

20. Intriguingly, a study in *Diabetes* in . . . : Schafer MJ, White TA, Evans G, et al. 'Exercise Prevents Diet-Induced Cellular Senescence in Adipose Tissue'. *Diabetes*. 2016;65(6):1606-1615.

20. The effects of using growth hormone . . . : Junnila RK, List EO, Berryman DE, Murrey JW, Kopchick JJ. 'The GH/IGF-1 axis in ageing and longevity'. *Nature Reviews Endocrinology*. 2013;9:366+.

21. Of the 300 people in the . . . : Laron Z. 'Lessons From 50 Years Of Study Of Laron Syndrome'. *Endocr Pract*. 2015;21(12):1395-1402.

Chapter 3: Ageing and the immune system

28. A key part of inflammation is . . . : Bäck M, Yurdagul A, Tabas I, Öörni K, Kovanen PT. 'Inflammation and its resolution in

atherosclerosis: mediators and therapeutic opportunities'. *Nature Reviews Cardiology*. 2019;16(7):389-406.

29. One theory is that the accumulation . . . : Franceschi C, Garagnani P, Parini P, Giuliani C, Santoro A. 'Inflammaging: a new immune–metabolic viewpoint for age-related diseases'. *Nature Reviews Endocrinology*. 2018;14(10):576-590.

29. Chronic infection, such as HIV, is . . . : Franceschi C, Campisi J. 'Chronic inflammation (inflammaging) and its potential contribution to age-associated disease's. *J Gerontol A Biol Sci Med Sci*. 2014;69 Suppl 1:S4-9.

30. This may be because the high . . . : Salvestrini V, Sell C, Lorenzini A. 'Obesity May Accelerate the Aging Process'. *Frontiers in Endocrinology*. 2019;10(266).

31. In the context of sauna, or . . . : Raison CL, Knight JM, Pariante C. 'Interleukin (IL)-6: A good kid hanging out with bad friends (and why sauna is good for health)'. *Brain Behav Immun*. 2018;73:1-2.

32. This is compared to 0.19 per cent . . . : ' Zhou F, Yu T, Du R, et al. 'Clinical course and risk factors for mortality of adult inpatients with COVID-19 in Wuhan, China: a retrospective cohort study'. *The Lancet*. 2020;395(10229):1054-1062.

33. This means that one of the . . . : Aiello A, Farzaneh F, Candore G, et al. 'Immunosenescence and Its Hallmarks: How to Oppose Aging Strategically? A Review of Potential Options for Therapeutic Intervention'. *Frontiers in Immunology*. 2019;10(2247).

Chapter 4: Ageing and gut health

37. Breastmilk also contains milk oligosaccharides, which . . . : Steven Townsend. 'Sugars in mother's milk help shape baby's microbiome and ward off infection'. *The Conversation*, https://theconversation.com/sugars-in-mothers-milk-help-shape-babys-microbiome-and-ward-off-infection-95746. Accessed.

38. Not surprisingly, this hasn't been as . . . : Vrieze A, Van Nood E, Holleman F, et al. 'Transfer of intestinal microbiota from lean donors increases insulin sensitivity in individuals with metabolic syndrome'. *Gastroenterology*. 2012;143(4):913-916.e917.

38. In a fascinating study led by . . . : Chambers ES, Viardot A, Psichas A, et al.' Effects of targeted delivery of propionate to the human colon on appetite regulation, body weight maintenance and adiposity in overweight adults'. *Gut*. 2015;64(11):1744.

40. In animal models, these have been . . . : Zhao J, Bi W, Xiao S, et al. 'Neuroinflammation induced by lipopolysaccharide causes cognitive impairment in mice'. *Scientific Reports*. 2019;9(1):5790.

40. Providing your microbes a good supply . . . : Camilleri M. 'Leaky gut: mechanisms, measurement and clinical implications in humans'. *Gut*. 2019;68(8):1516-1526.

41. Around 80–90 per cent of the fibres . . . : Berthoud HR, Neuhuber WL. 'Functional and chemical anatomy of the afferent vagal system'. *Auton Neurosci*. 2000;85(1-3):1-17.

42. The messages the vagus nerve carries back . . . : Breit S, Kupferberg A, Rogler G, Hasler G. 'Vagus Nerve as Modulator of the Brain-Gut Axis in Psychiatric and Inflammatory Disorders'. *Frontiers in Psychiatry*. 2018;9:44-44.

42. Many symbionts, aka friendly bacteria, actually . . . : Johnson KVA, Foster KR. 'Why does the microbiome affect behaviour?'. *Nature Reviews Microbiology*. 2018;16(10):647-655.

42. Some research has shown a link . . . : Kelly JR, Borre Y, C OB, et al. 'Transferring the blues: Depression-associated gut microbiota induces neurobehavioural changes in the rat'. *J Psychiatr Res*. 2016;82:109-118.

42. A 2019 study published in *Nature Microbiology* . . . : Valles-Colomer M, Falony G, Darzi Y, et al. 'The neuroactive potential of the human gut microbiota in quality of life and depression'. *Nature Microbiology*. 2019.

43. In one study, frail older adults who . . . : Claesson MJ, Jeffery IB, Conde S, et al. 'Gut microbiota composition correlates with diet and health in the elderly'. *Nature*. 2012;488(7410):178-184.

43. Other studies have looked at the . . . : Biagi E, Rampelli S, Turroni S, Quercia S, Candela M, Brigidi P. 'The gut microbiota of centenarians: Signatures of longevity in the gut microbiota profile'. *Mechanisms of Ageing and Development*. 2017;165:180-184.

44. In recent years, a new treatment . . . : Borody TJRS. 'Fecal microbiota transplantation for treatment of recurrent Clostridioides (formerly Clostridium) difficile infection'. *UpToDate*. 2019.

46. Studies of faecal samples from people . . . : Guyonnet D, Chassany O, Ducrotte P, et al. 'Effect of a fermented milk containing Bifidobacterium animalis DN-173 010 on the health-related quality of life and symptoms in irritable bowel syndrome in adults in primary care: a multicentre, randomized, double-blind, controlled trial'. *Aliment Pharmacol Ther*. 2007;26(3):475-486.

46. Researchers have also found that people . . . : Kok CR, Hutkins R. 'Yogurt and other fermented foods as sources of health-promoting bacteria'. *Nutr Rev*. 2018;76(Supplement_1):4-15.

47. Many bacteria are similar: they require . . . : Zapata HJ, Quagliarello VJ. 'The microbiota and microbiome in aging: potential implications in health and age-related diseases'. *J Am Geriatr Soc*. 2015;63(4):776-781.

Chapter 5: Ageing, stress and mental health

49. Severe stressful life events, such as . . . : Shah SM, Carey IM, Harris T, Dewilde S, Victor CR, Cook DG. 'The effect of unexpected bereavement on mortality in older couples'. *Am J Public Health*. 2013;103(6):1140-1145.

53: Cortisol levels have a diurnal variation . . . : Reddy TE, Pauli F, Sprouse RO, et al. 'Genomic determination of the glucocorticoid response reveals unexpected mechanisms of gene regulation'. *Genome Research*. 2009;19(12):2163-2171.

53. However, this negative feedback loop can . . . : Joëls M, Baram TZ. 'The neuro-symphony of stress'. *Nat Rev Neurosci*. 2009;10(6):459-466.

54. Cortisol can lead to increased abdominal . . . : van der Valk ES, Savas M, van Rossum EFC. 'Stress and Obesity: Are There More Susceptible Individuals?'. *Curr Obes Rep*. 2018;7(2):193-203.

54. The researcher found that a flat . . . : Hackett RA, Steptoe A, Kumari M.' Association of diurnal patterns in salivary cortisol with type 2 diabetes in the Whitehall II study'. *J Clin Endocrinol Metab*. 2014;99(12):4625-4631.

54. At follow-up, these people were slightly . . . : Hackett RA, Kivimaki M, Kumari M, Steptoe A. 'Diurnal Cortisol Patterns, Future Diabetes, and Impaired Glucose Metabolism in the Whitehall II Cohort Study'. *J Clin Endocrinol Metab*. 2016;101(2):619-625.

54. In the short term, cortisol can . . . : Hannibal KE, Bishop MD. 'Chronic stress, cortisol dysfunction, and pain: a psychoneuroendocrine rationale for stress management in pain rehabilitation'. *Physical Therapy*. 2014;94(12):1816-1825.

55. There is an association between high . . . : Mathur MB, Epel E, Kind S, et al. 'Perceived stress and telomere length: A systematic review, meta-analysis, and methodologic considerations for advancing the field'. *Brain Behav Immun*. 2016;54:158-169.

55. The city of Glasgow provides another . . . : Reid M. 'Behind the "Glasgow effect"'. *Bull World Health Organ*. 2011;89(10):706-707.

58. Fascinatingly, data from the Whitehall Study . . . : Gimeno D, Kivimäki M, Brunner EJ, et al. 'Associations of C-reactive protein and interleukin-6 with cognitive symptoms of depression: 12-year follow-up of the Whitehall II study'. *Psychological Medicine*. 2009;39(3):413-423.

62. Another evolving treatment for depression is . . . : Janssen CW, Lowry CA, Mehl MR, et al. 'Whole-Body Hyperthermia for the Treatment of Major Depressive Disorder: A Randomized Clinical Trial'. *JAMA Psychiatry*. 2016;73(8):789-795.

63. This complex action is because alcohol . . . : Vengeliene V, Bilbao A, Molander A, Spanagel R. 'Neuropharmacology of alcohol addiction'. *Br J Pharmacol*. 2008;154(2):299-315.

Chapter 6: The male–female longevity paradox

65. One reason for this is that . . . : *World Health Statistics 2016: Monitoring health for the SDGs Annex B: tables of health statistics by country, WHO region and globally.* Geneva, Switzerland, World Health Organisation, 2016.

65. Another is that although women live . . . : *Australian Bureau of Statistics (ABS) 2016. Survey of Disability, Ageing and Carers: Summary of Findings, 2015.* Canberra: ABS.

67. A study of three Siberian towns . . . : Zaridze D, Lewington S, Boroda A, et al. 'Alcohol and mortality in Russia: prospective observational study of 151 000 adults'. *The Lancet.* 2014;383(9927):1465-1473.

68. When there are two active copies . . . : Hubbard RE. 'Sex Differences in Frailty'. *Interdiscip Top Gerontol Geriatr.* 2015;41:41-53.

71. Women who have had children also . . . : Pollack AZ, Rivers K, Ahrens KA. 'Parity associated with telomere length among US reproductive age women'. *Hum Reprod.* 2018.

71. This is also balanced by the . . . : Bodelon C, Wentzensen N, Schonfeld SJ, et al. 'Hormonal risk factors and invasive epithelial ovarian cancer risk by parity'. *British Journal of Cancer.* 2013;109(3):769-776.

71. This is also balanced by the . . . : Lambe M, Hsieh CC, Chan HW, Ekbom A, Trichopoulos D, Adami HO. 'Parity, age at first and last birth, and risk of breast cancer: a population-based study in Sweden'. *Breast Cancer Res Treat.* 1996;38(3):305-311.

71–2. In a historical analysis of English . . . : Westendorp RGJ, Kirkwood TBL. 'Human longevity at the cost of reproductive success'. *Nature.* 1998;396:743.

72. Yet other recent longitudinal studies of . . . : *Reproduction later in life is a marker for longevity in women.* Science Daily. https://www.sciencedaily.com/releases/2014/06/140625101750.htm. Accessed 12th December, 2019.

73. In the Russian study referred to . . . : Oksuzyan A, Shkolnikova M, Vaupel JW, Christensen K, Shkolnikov VM. 'Sex Differences in Biological Markers of Health in the Study of Stress, Aging and Health in Russia'. *PLoS One.* 2015;10(6):e0131691.

73. Although cardiovascular disease is the leading . . . : Kuehn BM. 'State of the Heart for Women'. *Circulation.* 2019;139(8):1121-1123.

74. In Australia, women who retired in . . . : Clare R. 'Superannuation account balances by age and gender'. The Association of Superannuation Funds of Australia Limited (2017). https://www.superannuation.asn.au/ArticleDocuments/359/1710_Superannuation_account_balances_by_age_and_gender.pdf.aspx

75. This is not surprising when you . . . : *BLS Reports.* 'Highlights of women's earnings in 2018'. U.S. Bureau of Labor Statistics. 2019;1083.

Chapter 7: What is health?

79. A study of centenarians found that . . . : Evert J, Lawler E, Bogan H, Perls T. 'Morbidity Profiles of Centenarians: Survivors, Delayers, and Escapers'. *The Journals of Gerontology: Series A.* 2003;58(3):M232-M237.

80. Cigarette smoke is a mixture of . . . : Moktar A, Ravoori S, Vadhanam MV, Gairola CG, Gupta RC. 'Cigarette smoke-induced DNA damage and repair detected by the comet assay in HPV-transformed cervical cells'. *International journal of oncology.* 2009;35(6):1297-1304.

80. This means that smoking will increase . . . : Kojima G, Iliffe S, Walters K. 'Smoking as a predictor of frailty: a systematic review'. *BMC Geriatrics.* 2015;15:131-131.

Chapter 8: Nourishment

88. Observational studies have shown that in . . . : Levine Morgan E, Suarez Jorge A, Brandhorst S, et al. Low Protein Intake Is Associated with a Major Reduction in IGF-1, Cancer, and Overall Mortality in the 65 and Younger but Not Older Population. *Cell Metab.* 2014;19(3):407-417.

89. While some short-term studies show some . . . : Paoli A, Rubini A, Volek JS, Grimaldi KA. Beyond weight loss: a review of the therapeutic uses of very-low-carbohydrate (ketogenic) diets. *European journal of clinical nutrition.* 2013;67(8):789-796.

94. One of the best studied is . . . : Kouris-Blazos A, Itsiopoulos C. Low all-cause mortality despite high cardiovascular risk in elderly Greek-born Australians: attenuating potential of diet? *Asia Pac J Clin Nutr.* 2014;23(4):532-544.

94. In a study published in *The Lancet* . . . : Chambers ES, Byrne CS, Frost G. Carbohydrate and human health: is it all about quality? *The Lancet.* 2019;393(10170):384-386.

95. High intake of phenolic-rich fruits, vegetables . . . : Zhang H, Tsao R. 'Dietary polyphenols, oxidative stress and antioxidant and anti-inflammatory effects'. *Current Opinion in Food Science.* 2016;8:33-42.

95. Diets high in red meat may . . . : Jeyakumar A, Dissabandara L, Gopalan V. 'A critical overview on the biological and molecular features of red and processed meat in colorectal carcinogenesis'. *Journal of Gastroenterology.* 2017;52(4):407-418.

96. According to *Public Health Nutrition*, 'ultra-processed' . . . : Monteiro CA, Cannon G, Moubarac J-C, Levy RB, Louzada MLC, Jaime PC. 'The UN Decade of Nutrition, the NOVA food classification and the trouble with ultra-processing'. *Public Health Nutrition.* 2018;21(1):5-17.

97. In one trial, a group of . . . : Hall KD, Ayuketah A, Brychta R, et al. 'Ultra-Processed Diets Cause Excess Calorie Intake and Weight

Gain: An Inpatient Randomized Controlled Trial of Ad Libitum Food Intake'. *Cell Metab.* 2019;30(1):67-77.e63.

97. Similarly, even though most supermarkets do . . . : Lawrence MA, Baker PI.' Ultra-processed food and adverse health outcomes'. *BMJ.* 2019;365:l2289.

98. The actual numbers of deaths were . . . : Rico-Campà A, Martínez-González MA, Alvarez-Alvarez I, et al. 'Association between consumption of ultra-processed foods and all cause mortality: SUN prospective cohort study'. *BMJ.* 2019;365:l1949.

98. This study was published in the same . . . : Srour B, Fezeu LK, Kesse-Guyot E, et al. 'Ultra-processed food intake and risk of cardiovascular disease: prospective cohort study (NutriNet-Santé)'. *BMJ.* 2019;365:l1451.

98. Eating highly processed foods is also . . . : Tilg H, Moschen AR. 'Food, Immunity, and the Microbiome'. *Gastroenterology.* 2015;148(6):1107-1119.

99. In mice, this has been linked . . . : Chassaing B, Koren O, Goodrich JK, et al. 'Dietary emulsifiers impact the mouse gut microbiota promoting colitis and metabolic syndrome'. *Nature.* 2015;519 (7541):92-96.

99. This may partly explain the link . . . : Spencer SJ, Korosi A, Layé S, Shukitt-Hale B, Barrientos RM. 'Food for thought: how nutrition impacts cognition and emotion'. *npj Science of Food.* 2017;1(1):7.

100. Western diet performed worse on memory . . . : Stevenson RJ, Francis HM, Attuquayefio T, et al. 'Hippocampal-dependent appetitive control is impaired by experimental exposure to a Western-style diet'. *Royal Society Open Science.* 2020;7(2):191338.

101. After twelve weeks, the groups who . . . : Jacka FN, O'Neil A, Opie R, et al. 'A randomised controlled trial of dietary improvement for adults with major depression (the 'SMILES' trial)'. *BMC Med.* 2017;15(1):23.

102. It may be an advantage to . . . : Winter JE, MacInnis RJ, Wattanapenpaiboon N, Nowson CA. 'BMI and all-cause mortality in older adults: a meta-analysis'. *Am J Clin Nutr.* 2014;99(4):875-890.

106. Other animal studies found that fasting . . . : Longo VD, Panda S. 'Fasting, Circadian Rhythms, and Time-Restricted Feeding in Healthy Lifespan'. *Cell Metab.* 2016;23(6):1048-1059.

Chapter 9: Movement

112. Large epidemiological studies have shown again . . . : Lee IM, Shiroma EJ, Lobelo F, et al. 'Effect of physical inactivity on major non-communicable diseases worldwide: an analysis of burden of disease and life expectancy'. *The Lancet.* 2012;380(9838):219-229.

112. A study published in the *British Medical Journal* . . . : Badley E. 'Inactivity, disability, and death are all interlinked'. *BMJ*. 2014;348:g2804.

113. Exercise influences cellular ageing by creating . . . : de Sousa CV, Sales MM, Rosa TS, Lewis JE, de Andrade RV, Simoes HG. 'The Antioxidant Effect of Exercise: A Systematic Review and Meta-Analysis'. *Sports Med*. 2017;47(2):277-293.

114. One fascinating study published in *Cell Metabolism* . . . : Robinson MM, Dasari S, Konopka AR, et al. 'Enhanced Protein Translation Underlies Improved Metabolic and Physical Adaptations to Different Exercise Training Modes in Young and Old Humans'. *Cell Metab*. 2017;25(3):581-592.

114. In a study of 68 people . . . : Puterman E, Weiss J, Lin J, et al. 'Aerobic exercise lengthens telomeres and reduces stress in family caregivers: A randomized controlled trial - Curt Richter Award Paper 2018'. *Psychoneuroendocrinology*. 2018;98:245-252.

114. Exercise also has a striking effect . . . : Brown WMC, Davison GW, McClean CM, Murphy MH. 'A Systematic Review of the Acute Effects of Exercise on Immune and Inflammatory Indices in Untrained Adults'. *Sports medicine - open*. 2015;1(1):35-35.

115. Many large studies have shown that . . . : Wen CP, Wai JP, Tsai MK, et al. 'Minimum amount of physical activity for reduced mortality and extended life expectancy: a prospective cohort study'. *The Lancet*. 2011;378(9798):1244-1253.

116. In an 8.5-year study of 6622 . . . : Samieri C, Perier M, Gaye B, et al. 'Association of cardiovascular health level in older age with cognitive decline and incident dementia'. *JAMA*. 2018;320(7):657-664.

116. A study published in *Neurology* in . . . ; Hörder H, Johansson L, Guo X, et al. 'Midlife cardiovascular fitness and dementia'. *Neurology*. 2018.

116. Exercise also improves brain plasticity, which . . . : Hayes S, Hayes J, Cadden M, Verfaellie M. 'A review of cardiorespiratory fitness-related neuroplasticity in the aging brain'. *Frontiers in Aging Neuroscience*. 2013;5(31).

117. A study of 41 people with . . . : Colcombe SJ, Kramer AF, Erickson KI, et al. 'Cardiovascular fitness, cortical plasticity, and aging'. *Proc Natl Acad Sci U S A*. 2004;101(9):3316-3321.

117. The likely reason for all these . . . : Kandola A, Hendrikse J, Lucassen PJ, Yücel M. 'Aerobic Exercise as a Tool to Improve Hippocampal Plasticity and Function in Humans: Practical Implications for Mental Health Treatment'. *Frontiers in Human Neuroscience*. 2016;10:373-373.

118. Many studies have shown that an . . . : Herring MP, O'Connor PJ, Dishman RK. 'The Effect of Exercise Training on Anxiety Symptoms

Among Patients: A Systematic Review Exercise Training and Anxiety Symptoms'. *JAMA Internal Medicine*. 2010;170(4):321-331.

118. These can reduce anxiety, as well . . . : Sher L. 'Exercise, wellbeing, and endogenous molecules of mood'. *The Lancet*. 1996;348(9025):477.

118. Part of the reason exercise is . . . : Anderson E, Shivakumar G. 'Effects of exercise and physical activity on anxiety'. *Frontiers in Psychiatry*. 2013;4:27-27.

118. There used to be concerns that . . . : Watson SL, Weeks BK, Weis LJ, Harding AT, Horan SA, Beck BR. 'High-Intensity Resistance and Impact Training Improves Bone Mineral Density and Physical Function in Postmenopausal Women With Osteopenia and Osteoporosis: The LIFTMOR Randomized Controlled Trial'. *J Bone Miner Res*. 2018;33(2):211-220.

119. There is even evidence that these . . . : Kemmler W, von Stengel S. 'Bone: High-intensity exercise to prevent fractures – risk or gain?'. *Nat Rev Endocrinol*. 2018;14(1):6-8.

119. A 2019 study of 315,059 people . . . : Saint-Maurice PF, Coughlan D, Kelly SP, et al. 'Association of Leisure-Time Physical Activity Across the Adult Life Course With All-Cause and Cause-Specific Mortality'. *JAMA Network Open*. 2019;2(3):e190355-e190355.

120. Data from the Australian Bureau of Statistics . . . : *Australia's health 2018*. Canberra: AIHW: Australian Institute of Health and Welfare 2018.;2018.

122. One effective option is high intensity . . . :Milanović Z, Sporiš G, Weston M. 'Effectiveness of High-Intensity Interval Training (HIT) and Continuous Endurance Training for VO2max Improvements: A Systematic Review and Meta-Analysis of Controlled Trials'. *Sports Medicine*. 2015;45(10):1469-1481.

123. One study in older men showed . . . : Hikida RS, Staron RS, Hagerman FC, et al. 'Effects of high-intensity resistance training on untrained older men. II. Muscle fiber characteristics and nucleo-cytoplasmic relationships'. *J Gerontol A Biol Sci Med Sci*. 2000;55(7):B347-354.

124. In one meta-analysis (a summary . . . : Lomas-Vega R, Obrero-Gaitan E, Molina-Ortega FJ, Del-Pino-Casado R. 'Tai Chi for Risk of Falls. A Meta-analysis'. *J Am Geriatr Soc*. 2017;65(9):2037-2043.

124–25. A study of older women enrolled . . . : Viljoen JE, Christie CJ. 'The change in motivating factors influencing commencement, adherence and retention to a supervised resistance training programme in previously sedentary post-menopausal women: a prospective cohort study'. *BMC Public Health*. 2015;15:236.

Chapter 10: Sleep

134. Being sleep deprived can alter this . . . : Leproult R, Copinschi G, Buxton O, Van Cauter E. 'Sleep loss results in an elevation of cortisol levels the next evening'. *Sleep*. 1997;20(10):865-870.

135. Sleep doesn't just alter how your . . . : Spiegel K, Leproult R, Van Cauter E. 'Impact of sleep debt on metabolic and endocrine function'. *The Lancet*. 1999;354(9188):1435-1439.

136. Shift workers also suffer the adverse . . . : Gu F, Han J, Laden F, et al. 'Total and cause-specific mortality of U.S. nurses working rotating night shifts'. *Am J Prev Med*. 2015;48(3):241-252.

137. When you consider the impact of . . . : Cordone S, Annarumma L, Rossini PM, De Gennaro L. 'Sleep and β-Amyloid Deposition in Alzheimer Disease: Insights on Mechanisms and Possible Innovative Treatments'. *Front Pharmacol*. 2019;10:695-695.

137. In a study published in *Science* . . . : Fultz NE, Bonmassar G, Setsompop K, et al. 'Coupled electrophysiological, hemodynamic, and cerebrospinal fluid oscillations in human sleep'. *Science*. 2019;366(6465):628-631.

137. In another study, this time in humans . . . : Lim ASP, Kowgier M, Yu L, Buchman AS, Bennett DA. 'Sleep Fragmentation and the Risk of Incident Alzheimer's Disease and Cognitive Decline in Older Persons'. *Sleep*. 2013;36(7):1027-1032.

138. The weight of evidence definitely supports . . . : Lim MM, Gerstner JR, Holtzman DM. 'The sleep–wake cycle and Alzheimer's disease: what do we know?'. *Neurodegenerative Disease Management*. 2014;4(5):351-362.

138. In 434 adults who were part . . . : Jackowska M, Hamer M, Carvalho LA, Erusalimsky JD, Butcher L, Steptoe A. 'Short sleep duration is associated with shorter telomere length in healthy men: findings from the Whitehall II cohort study'. *PLoS One*. 2012;7(10):e47292.

138. In another study where most participants . . . : Prather AA, Hecht FM, Epel ES. 'Factors related to telomere length'. *Brain Behav Immun*. 2016;53:279.

140. Many of the sleep issues experienced . . . : Li J, Vitiello MV, Gooneratne NS. 'Sleep in Normal Aging'. *Sleep Medicine Clinics*. 2018;13(1):1-11.

142. Over the long term, the use . . . : He Q, Chen X, Wu T, Li L, Fei X. 'Risk of Dementia in Long-Term Benzodiazepine Users: Evidence from a Meta-Analysis of Observational Studies'. *J Clin Neurol*. 2019;15(1):9-19.

146. This can feel cruel if you . . . : Kyle SD, Miller CB, Rogers Z, Siriwardena AN, Macmahon KM, Espie CA. 'Sleep restriction therapy for insomnia is associated with reduced objective total sleep time, increased daytime somnolence, and objectively impaired vigilance:

implications for the clinical management of insomnia disorder'. *Sleep*. 2014;37(2):229-237.

Chapter 11: Challenging your brain

150. Executive function is negatively affected by . . . : Diamond A. 'Executive functions'. *Annual Review of Psychology*. 2013;64:135-168.
150. 'Declarative (explicit) memory is conscious recollection...': Harada CN, Natelson Love MC, Triebel KL. 'Normal cognitive aging'. *Clin Geriatr Med*. 2013;29(4):737-752.
152. Worryingly, there is evidence that retirement . . . : Meng A, Nexø MA, Borg V. 'The impact of retirement on age related cognitive decline – a systematic review'. *BMC Geriatrics*. 2017;17(1):160-160.
152. However, sometimes the decline may be . . . : Andel R, Infurna FJ, Hahn Rickenbach EA, Crowe M, Marchiondo L, Fisher GG. 'Job strain and trajectories of change in episodic memory before and after retirement: results from the Health and Retirement Study'. *J Epidemiol Community Health*. 2015;69(5):442-446.
155. By quietening the mind, meditation can . . . : Schöne B, Gruber T, Graetz S, Bernhof M, Malinowski P. 'Mindful breath awareness meditation facilitates efficiency gains in brain networks: A steady-state visually evoked potentials study'. *Scientific Reports*. 2018;8(1):13687.
155. Research has shown that meditation can . . . : Luders E, Cherbuin N, Kurth F. 'Forever Young(er): potential age-defying effects of long-term meditation on gray matter atrophy'. *Front Psychol*. 2015;5:1551-1551.
156. Meditation also lowers the physiological effects . . . : Rosenkranz MA, Davidson RJ, Maccoon DG, Sheridan JF, Kalin NH, Lutz A.' A comparison of mindfulness-based stress reduction and an active control in modulation of neurogenic inflammation'. *Brain Behav Immun*. 2013;27(1):174-184.
157. In one of the larger studies . . . : Owen AM, Hampshire A, Grahn JA, et al. 'Putting brain training to the test'. *Nature*. 2010;465:775.
157. In one of the earlier trials . . . : Rebok GW, Ball K, Guey LT, et al. 'Ten-year effects of the advanced cognitive training for independent and vital elderly cognitive training trial on cognition and everyday functioning in older adults'. *Journal of the American Geriatrics Society*. 2014;62(1):16-24.
160. While higher levels of education are . . . : Vemuri P, Lesnick TG, Przybelski SA, et al. 'Association of lifetime intellectual enrichment with cognitive decline in the older population'. *JAMA Neurol*. 2014;71(8):1017-1024.

Chapter 12: Connection

163. Sharing an experience with another person . . . : Wagner U, Galli L, Schott BH, et al. 'Beautiful friendship: Social sharing of emotions improves subjective feelings and activates the neural reward circuitry'. *Social cognitive and affective neuroscience.* 2015;10(6):801-808.

165. Studies have shown that people with . . . : Rafnsson SB, Orrell M, d'Orsi E, Hogervorst E, Steptoe A. 'Loneliness, Social Integration, and Incident Dementia Over 6 Years: Prospective Findings From the English Longitudinal Study of Ageing'. *The Journals of Gerontology: Series B.* 2017;75(1):114-124.

165. People who are lonely have a . . . : Jaremka LM, Fagundes CP, Peng J, et al. 'Loneliness promotes inflammation during acute stress'. *Psychol Sci.* 2013;24(7):1089-1097.

165. Loneliness even impacts sleep . . . : Cacioppo JT, Hawkley LC, Crawford LE, et al. 'Loneliness and health: potential mechanisms'. *Psychosom Med.* 2002;64(3):407-417.

167. Socialising helps regulate immune function . . . : Heffner KL, Waring ME, Roberts MB, Eaton CB, Gramling R. 'Social isolation, C-reactive protein, and coronary heart disease mortality among community-dwelling adults'. *Soc Sci Med.* 2011;72(9):1482-1488.

167. The Midlife in the US study . . . : Seeman TE, Miller-Martinez DM, Stein Merkin S, Lachman ME, Tun PA, Karlamangla AS. 'Histories of social engagement and adult cognition: midlife in the U.S. study'. *The Journals of Gerontology Series B.* 2011;66 Suppl 1(Suppl 1):i141-i152.

170. Marriage has historically been better for . . . : Ploubidis GB, Silverwood RJ, DeStavola B, Grundy E.' Life-Course Partnership Status and Biomarkers in Midlife: Evidence From the 1958 British Birth Cohort'. *Am J Public Health.* 2015;105(8):1596-1603.

171. People who are married aren't just . . . : Umberson D, Williams K, Powers DA, Liu H, Needham B. 'You make me sick: marital quality and health over the life course'. *Journal of Health and Social Behavior.* 2006;47(1):1-16.

171. People who are married aren't just . . . : Monin JKC, M.S. 'Why Do Men Benefit More from Marriage Than Do Women? Thinking More Broadly About Interpersonal Processes That Occur Within and Outside of Marriage'. *Sex Roles.* 2011;65.

171. With the level of stress that . . . : Becker C, Kirchmaier I, Trautmann ST. 'Marriage, parenthood and social network: Subjective well-being and mental health in old age'. *PLOS ONE.* 2019;14(7):e0218704.

172. Caring for grandchildren isn't just . . . : Hilbrand S, Coall DA, Gerstorf D, Hertwig R. 'Caregiving within and beyond the family is associated with lower mortality for the caregiver: A prospective study'. *Evolution and Human Behavior.* 2017;38(3):397-403.

172. Data from the Australian Longitudinal Study ... : Tooth L LD, Chan H, Coombe J, Dobson A, Hockey R, Townsend N, Byles J & Mishra G. *From child care to elder care: Findings from the Australian Longitudinal Study on Women's Health*. Report prepared for the Australian Government Department of Health; May 2018, 2018.

173. Regularly spending time with grandchildren is ... : Flouri E, Buchanan A, Tan JP, Griggs J, Attar-Schwartz S. 'Adverse life events, area socio-economic disadvantage, and adolescent psychopathology: The role of closeness to grandparents in moderating the effect of contextual stress'. *Stress*. 2010;13(5):402-412.

174. In a study in England, 14 per cent ... : Durcan DBR. *Local action on health inequalities - Reducing social isolation across the lifecourse*. London: Public Health England; 2015.

174. In Australia, men aged 85 and ... : Australian Bureau of Statistics. (2019). *Intentional self harm key characteristics*. Accessed 1 October, 2019.

Chapter 13: Nurturing wellbeing

179. In a multi-country study people were ... : Falk H, Skoog I, Johansson L, et al. 'Self-rated health and its association with mortality in older adults in China, India and Latin America—a 10/66 Dementia Research Group study'. *Age and Ageing*. 2017;46(6):932-939.

180. People in the former Soviet Union ... : Steptoe A, Deaton A, Stone AA. 'Subjective wellbeing, health, and ageing'. *The Lancet*. 2015;385(9968):640-648.

181. In one study conducted by The Women's Health Initiative ... : Tindle HA, Chang Y-F, Kuller LH, et al. 'Optimism, cynical hostility, and incident coronary heart disease and mortality in the Women's Health Initiative'. *Circulation*. 2009;120(8):656-662.

182. In a study of 2280 men ... : Ikeda A, Schwartz J, Peters JL, et al. 'Optimism in relation to inflammation and endothelial dysfunction in older men: the VA Normative Aging Study'. *Psychosom Med*. 2011;73(8):664-671.

182. Research suggests that it contributes ... : Ryff CD. 'The Benefits of Purposeful Life Engagement on Later-Life Physical Function'. *JAMA Psychiatry*. 2017;74(10):1046-1047.

183. One study measured levels of purpose ... : Zilioli S, Slatcher RB, Ong AD, Gruenewald TL. 'Purpose in life predicts allostatic load ten years later'. *Journal of Psychosomatic Research*. 2015;79(5):451-457.

183. One of the most interesting studies ... : Boyle PA, Buchman AS, Wilson RS, Yu L, Schneider JA, Bennett DA. 'Effect of purpose in life on the relation between Alzheimer disease pathologic changes on cognitive function in advanced age'. *Archives of General Psychiatry*. 2012;69(5):499-505.

184. Some strategies for developing purpose can . . . : Beth Kurland. *How to Create Meaning and Purpose in Our Daily Lives.* https://www.psychologytoday.com/au/blog/the-well-being-toolkit/201810/how-create-meaning-and-purpose-in-our-daily-lives. Published 2018. Accessed 11 October, 2019.

184. In a study led by Professor Becca Levy . . . : Levy BR, Slade MD, Pietrzak RH, Ferrucci L. 'Positive age beliefs protect against dementia even among elders with high-risk gene'. *PLOS ONE.* 2018;13(2):e0191004.

185. In another analysis of this cohort . . . : Levy BR, Bavishi A. 'Survival Advantage Mechanism: Inflammation as a Mediator of Positive Self-Perceptions of Aging on Longevity'. *The Journals of Gerontology: Series B.* 2016;73(3):409-412.

186. However, botox also acts on the . . . : Davis JI, Senghas A, Brandt F, Ochsner KN. 'The Effects of BOTOX® Injections on Emotional Experience'. *Emotion (Washington, DC).* 2010;10(3):433-440.

187. People who are navigating loss have . . . : McGrath P, Holewa H, McNaught M. 'Surviving spousal bereavement Insights for GPs'. *Australian Family Physician.* 2010;39:780-783.

187. Many older adults actually have high . . . : MacLeod S, Musich S, Hawkins K, Alsgaard K, Wicker ER. 'The impact of resilience among older adults'. *Geriatr Nurs.* 2016;37(4):266-272.

189. Some researchers have looked at . . . : Redwine LS, Henry BL, Pung MA, et al. 'Pilot Randomized Study of a Gratitude Journaling Intervention on Heart Rate Variability and Inflammatory Biomarkers in Patients With Stage B Heart Failure'. *Psychosom Med.* 2016;78(6):667-676.

Chapter 14: Making change

193. In a study led by Professor Linda Fried . . . : Hong SI, Morrow-Howell N. 'Health outcomes of Experience Corps: a high-commitment volunteer program'. *Soc Sci Med.* 2010;71(2):414-420.

Chapter 15: Dementia

209. Another theory postulates that dementia . . . : Ferreira LSS, Fernandes CS, Vieira MNN, De Felice FG. 'Insulin Resistance in Alzheimer's Disease'. *Frontiers in Neuroscience.* 2018;12:830-830.

210. Professor Ruth Itzhaki of Oxford University . . . : Itzhaki RF. 'Corroboration of a Major Role for Herpes Simplex Virus Type 1 in Alzheimer's Disease'. *Frontiers in Aging Neuroscience.* 2018;10(324).

210. On MRI we can see 'white matter hyperintensities' . . . : Merino JG. 'White Matter Hyperintensities on Magnetic Resonance Imaging: What Is a Clinician to Do?'. *Mayo Clinic Proceedings.* 2019;94(3):380-382.

217. The original randomised trial included people with . . . : Reisberg

B, Doody R, Stöffler A, Schmitt F, Ferris S, Möbius HJ. 'Memantine in Moderate-to-Severe Alzheimer's Disease'. *New England Journal of Medicine*. 2003;348(14):1333-1341.

220. A 2016 study showed that in the USA . . . : Langa KM, Larson EB, Crimmins EM, et al. 'A Comparison of the Prevalence of Dementia in the United States in 2000 and 2012Prevalence of Dementia in the United States in 2000 and 2012Prevalence of Dementia in the United States in 2000 and 2012'. *JAMA Internal Medicine*. 2017;177(1):51-58.

220. There are similar findings in the UK.: Ahmadi-Abhari S, Guzman-Castillo M, Bandosz P, et al. 'Temporal trend in dementia incidence since 2002 and projections for prevalence in England and Wales to 2040: modelling study'. *BMJ*. 2017;358:j2856.

221. Even for people who have two . . . : Solomon A, Turunen H, Ngandu T, et al. 'Effect of the Apolipoprotein E Genotype on Cognitive Change During a Multidomain Lifestyle Intervention: A Subgroup Analysis of a Randomized Clinical Trial'. *JAMA Neurol*. 2018;75(4):462-470.

Chapter 16: Fraility

223. The medical definition of frailty is . . . : Clegg A, Young J, Iliffe S, Rikkert MO, Rockwood K. 'Frailty in elderly people'. *The Lancet*. 2013;381(9868):752-762.

227. However, the relationship only works in . . . : Kleipool EE, Hoogendijk EO, Trappenburg MC, et al. 'Frailty in Older Adults with Cardiovascular Disease: Cause, Effect or Both?'. *Aging Dis*. 2018;9(3):489-497.

227. One study published in 2018 demonstrated . . . : Xu M, Pirtskhalava T, Farr JN, et al. 'Senolytics improve physical function and increase lifespan in old age'. *Nature Medicine*. 2018;24(8):1246-1256.

228. People who are frail tend to have . . . : Li H, Manwani B, Leng SX. 'Frailty, inflammation, and immunity'. *Aging Dis*. 2011;2(6):466-473.

230. A fascinating clue to the way frailty . . . : Wang C, Song X, Mitnitski A, et al. 'Effect of health protective factors on health deficit accumulation and mortality risk in older adults in the Beijing Longitudinal Study of Aging'. *J Am Geriatr Soc*. 2014;62(5):821-828.

Chpater 17: Heart disease

240. In 2017 the American Heart Association . . . : Davis E, Gorog DA, Rihal C, Prasad A, Srinivasan M. '"Mind the gap" acute coronary syndrome in women: A contemporary review of current clinical evidence'. *Int J Cardiol*. 2017;227:840-849.

241. In a study from Florida, women . . . : Greenwood BN, Carnahan S, Huang L. 'Patient-physician gender concordance and increased

mortality among female heart attack patients'. *Proc Natl Acad Sci U S A*. 2018;115(34):8569-8574.

Chapter 18: Stroke

245. Stroke is the eighth leading cause . . . : Health AIo, Welfare. *Stroke and its management in Australia: an update*. Canberra: AIHW;2013.

246. As with an AMI, knowing the symptoms of stroke . . . : Stroke Foundation. https://strokefoundation.org.au/About-Stroke/Stroke-symptoms. Accessed 12 November, 2019.

Chapter 19: Diabetes

251. The UKPDS study recruited people . . . : 'Intensive blood-glucose control with sulphonylureas or insulin compared with conventional treatment and risk of complications in patients with type 2 diabetes (UKPDS 33)'. *The Lancet*. 1998;352(9131):837-853.

252. In 2008, another study was published . . . : 'Effects of Intensive Glucose Lowering in Type 2 Diabetes'. *New England Journal of Medicine*. 2008;358(24):2545-2559.

253. In a study of over 5000 people . . . . : Gregg EW, Chen H, Wagenknecht LE, et al. 'Association of an intensive lifestyle intervention with remission of type 2 diabetes'. *Jama*. 2012;308(23):2489-2496.

253. Both time-restricted eating and a 4:3 regime . . . . : de Cabo R, Mattson MP. 'Effects of Intermittent Fasting on Health, Aging, and Disease'. *New England Journal of Medicine*. 2019;381(26):2541-2551.

Chapter 20: Cancer

258. Since breast screening was introduced in 1991 . . . : Burton RC, Bell RJ, Thiagarajah G, Stevenson C. 'Adjuvant therapy, not mammographic screening, accounts for most of the observed breast cancer specific mortality reductions in Australian women since the national screening program began in 1991'. *Breast Cancer Research and Treatment*. 2012;131(3):949-955.

Chapter 21: Musculoskeletal disorders

266–67. It's falling from standing height, which . . . : Beck B, Cameron P, Lowthian J, Fitzgerald M, Judson R, Gabbe BJ. 'Major trauma in older persons'. *BJS Open*. 2018;2(5):310-318.

268. While calcium and vitamin D play . . . : Bolland MJ, Avenell A, Baron JA, et al. 'Effect of calcium supplements on risk of myocardial infarction and cardiovascular events: meta-analysis'. *BMJ*. 2010;341:c3691.

INDEX